SAVAGE

BODYWORK

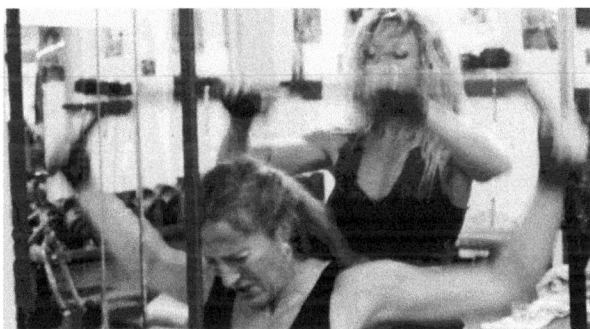

LY DE ANGELES
—LORE—

SAVAGE – BODYWORK

Health, nutrition, resistance training wildcraft wisdom and a touch of witch

1st Edition 2023

Updated and expanded from Body Language.

ISBN 9780645521443

(2023)

Cover design   LOÐBRÓKSIGURÐ

Cover Photography – Donatella Parisini

OTHER BOOKS BY THE AUTHOR

Witchcraft Theory and Practice, Llewellyn, USA, 2000

When I See the Wild God, Llewellyn, USA, 2002

Pagan Visions for a Sustainable Future, Llewellyn, USA, 2004

The Quickening, Book 1 of the Traveler Series, Llewellyn, USA, 2005

The Shining Isle, Book 2 of the Traveler Series, Llewellyn, USA, 2006

Tarot Theory and Practice, Llewellyn, USA, 2007

Magdalene | Witch of the Grail Legends, Australia, USA, 2012

Genesis | The Future, Australia, USA, revised edition, 2012

The Feast of Flesh and Spirit, Interstitial, Australia, USA, 2013

Priteni | *The Decimation of the Indigenous Britons*. Australia, USA, 2015

Initiation | *A Memoir*, Australia, USA, 2016

The Skellig | *A Shapeshifter Tale*, Australia, USA, 2017

Witch | *For Those Who Are*, Australia, USA, 2018

Under Snow, Book 3 of the Traveler Series, co-authored by Serenity de Angeles, Australia, 2019

Advanced Tarot | *The Voyage of Prophecy*, Australia, USA, 2020

Brave | *For the Unclaimed People,* Australia, USA, 2021

The Changeling | *From Winter, Spring is Born,* Book 4 of the Traveler Series, Australia, USA, 2022, now also available in audiobook format at Bandcamp[1]

---

[1]https://lydeangeles.bandcamp.com/album/the-changeling-from-winter-spring-is-born-magical-realism

ADVICE

This book is based on personal experience, opinion and research. I am not affiliated with any institution, corporation or organization, and neither do I hold traditionally accepted academic letters, on this subject, after my name. I am, in any discussion of martial arts, an accredited 3rd Dan Iaido instructor.

CONTENTS

___

FOOD

HEY TRICKSTER, NOT SORRY

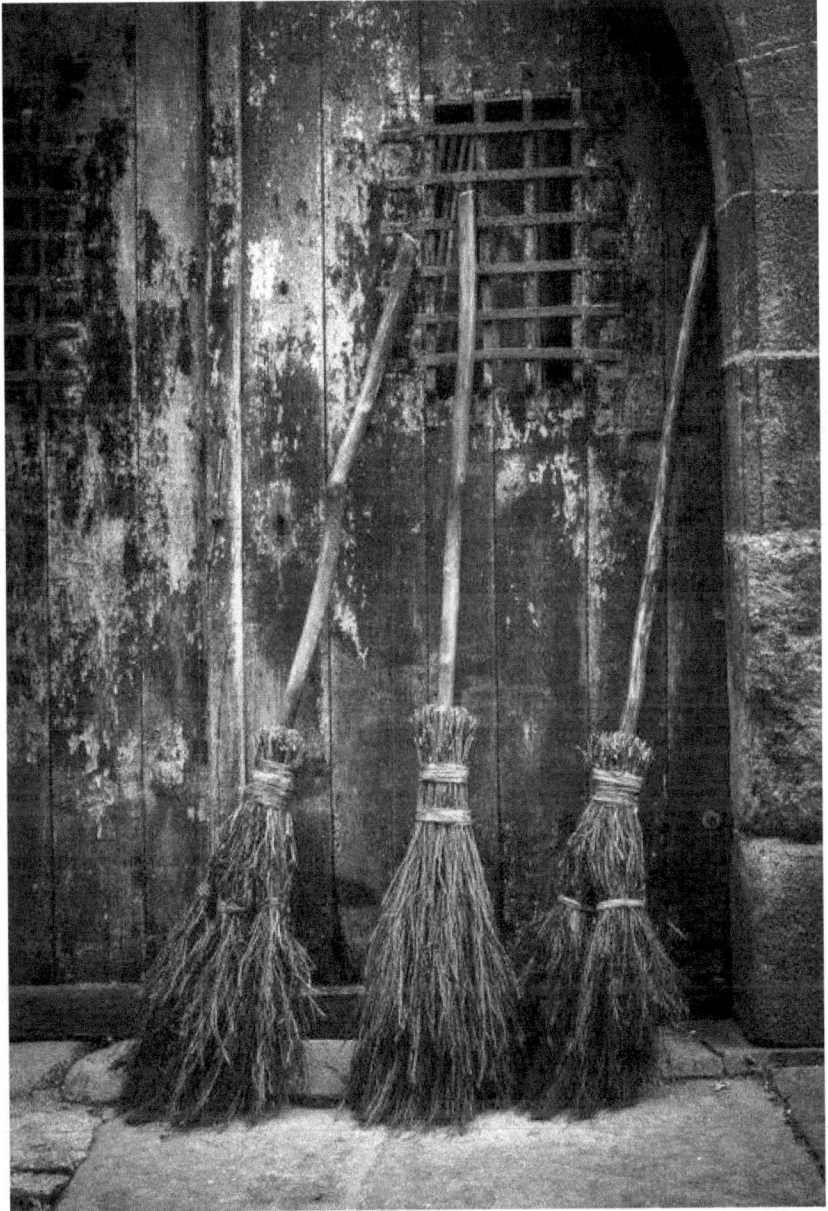

SAVAGE begins here…

Mother Earth,
Enlighten what's dark in
me,
Strengthen what's weak
in me,
Mend what's broken in
me,
Heal what's sick in me,
And lastly,
Revive whatever peace
and love has died in me.

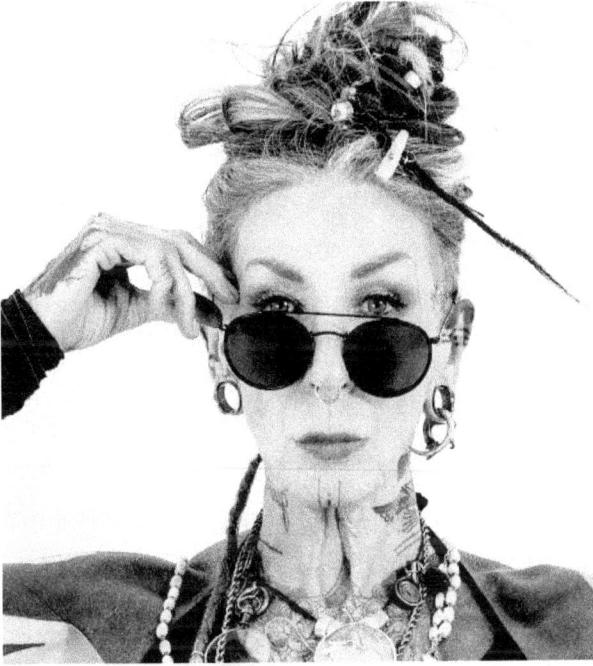

Ly de Angeles – Lore – 2022

I KNOW WOMEN

When we look into a mirror we seek flaws. In our faces we see lines or open pores or dry skin or broken capillaries; we see a nose too big or too pointed; chins that sag or bags beneath tired eyes. In body we see thighs too fat, too droopy, too big; waists and bottoms that are never right; wobbly upper arms; love-handles that are hidden beneath long tee-shirts—and always we secretly or fearfully talk about what we ought to do about it, despairing and casually embarrassed.

Ask yourself, you who see these things and sense distress: Why do I see myself so? Ask yourself whether the secret condemnation you feel about your physical form is of your own making?

You give of your strength and compassion to the world around you every day. You strive to meet the challenges and responsibilities of merely living. You suppress the urge to desert your kids. To have sex with strangers. Maybe. Sometimes? You make a difference to the way the world is.

Do you compare yourself to others? Do you compromise your choices because someone thinks you're *too* something? Do you yearn to be loved? Honored for your worth? Respected for no reason other than that you are fabulously alive? To feel good about—fill in the dots? To be really liked? And do you feel that only someone else can make things better for you? Oh, what lies we've let ourselves believe.

We can be merciless upon ourselves for not fitting *someone else's* idea of what is acceptably beautiful.

And yet, ask yourself: Who defines our concept of beauty?

As a psychic, counsellor, questioner, creative, witch, medicine woman yes, and body builder, I have listened to the blues being sung by thousands of women and girls over decades. They so often feel that they're not good enough. They blame it on, first and foremost, themselves, then the media, or men, or fashion, or modern western society. Or other women.

Someone ask me who defines the concept.

Go on, someone ask me.

I do.

It took me over forty years to be certain that I understood. I learned about the truth of things when I decided to do exactly what I wanted with my life; when I decided that it's *me* who should like the way I look. When I decided that I would never lie to myself about my motives in any matter, no matter what the repercussions. When I determined never to have to *try* to have someone like who I am.

I look at the Earth with her ragged mountains and her deep gorges; her canyons, her caves, her forests, her seas and her rivers, her vast tracts of desert, and my body is that. I know my moods of thunder and lightning, intolerable winds, hazy, smoky autumn evenings, days of grey stillness, hot and sweaty mid-summer afternoons, and the times when I'm ice on the water tank. I've got scars and stretch-marks and muscles on a tiny woman-body; I've got wrinkles from too much sun or too little back-up in times of trouble; a mane of hair that knows no comb – and, yes again, attitude.

I am Earth. I feel her, and we're the same. We are her mirror.

We are her mirrors. Do you understand now? Do you recognize yourself among all the people you try to be, for all the others you try to be someone for? You see, I've worked it out. It's not *what* you do in life that matters, or even who you are, but *that* you are. That's the important thing. To understand that is to set yourself free to know that everything that you say and do is an expression of you that you share with life itself.

I have trained women (and many men) in the art of bodywork for several years now. Some of their faces are amongst these photographs—

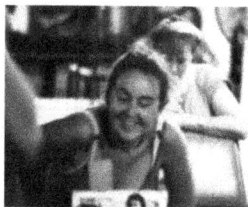

Tamara

Look at them. They love what they are doing. They love the differences they are making to their physical expression of who they are.

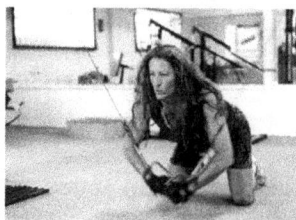

Cate

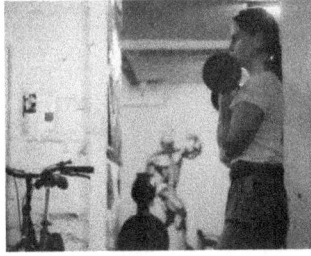

Kaye

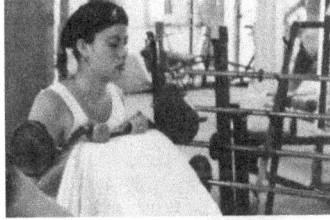

Milo

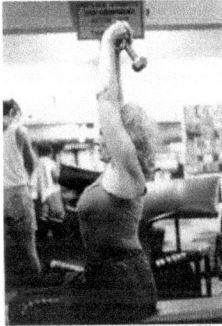

Virginia

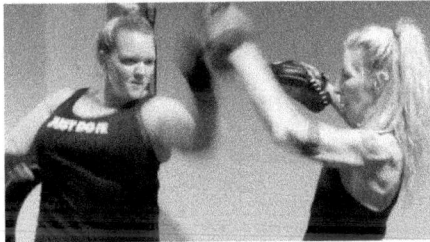

Caitlyn and Ly

We don't do this for competition. We don't do it to attract a lover or a spouse. We don't do it because it's trendy. We do it because it feels good. It's what we do to give ourselves pleasure.

You can look at the photos and think that maybe one or two of us are too fat or too thin, too muscly or too flabby, too old or too young. And you'd be wrong. Because there's that snippety little dismissive *too* (of which you will read later).

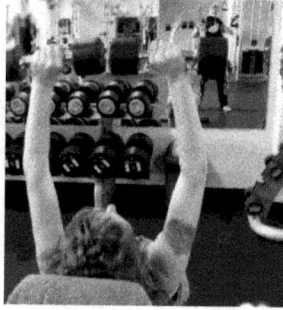

Nila

The strain, the pain, the challenge, the earthy sweaty grace? What you are seeing is beauty.

ON LEAVING 70

I write this workbook at the very close of 2022. I departed Melbourne—called Naarm by the people of the Kulin Nations—after ten years' study (extant), work and language exploration. And returned to the north. To Bunjalung country of the Arakwal Nation where I now complete this edition.

A few months before I left I fulfilled an odd dream prophesy I'd had as a kid. I dreamed healers had the technology to laser a body open if we were feeling unwell, and to spread us out like a map, checking our vital organs, sinew, bone, blood and anything else—that illogically didn't pour all over the examination table—find the glitch that made us feel unhealthy, fix it or replace it then roll us back into 3D again, lasering the opening and leaving no mark.

So it was out of curiosity when, in my seventieth year and after a fitness and nutritional regime that I had been honing for decades, I asked a physician for a referral to have all my organs ultra-sounded.

A week after this non-invasive, if somewhat slimy procedure I phoned for the results. The receptionist said *Oh, I have them here on screen. You're normal.* Of course I asked whether normal means healthy. They said *Seems so. No, visceral fat. No fatty liver. No stones in the gall bladder, kidneys or anywhere else.*

I responded, *it'll be something else that kills me, then, I suppose.*

...

Dear Diary,

I'm gonna turn this book to rags before my hand slaps the mat because...

(First published in *Archer Magazine*, 2017[2])

Hey Loki…

MISTER TRICKSTER…please explain.

How do I do what you want me to do?

How do I behave like you think I should?

How am I to be both me *and* age gracefully?

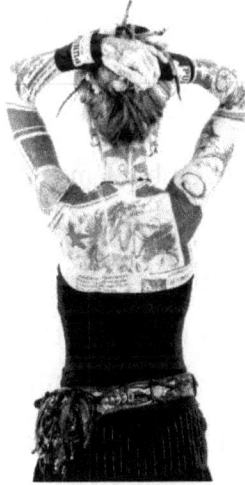

INK—Chauvet Cave Art, 40,000 years, France

AUTHENTICITY

As a healer and a seeker of authenticity I communicate with bodies, human and otherkin. To do this I first explore what works and what does not. Magic is, after all, both an art and a science.

[2] https://archermagazine.com.au/2018/06/shame-gender-ageing/

While others write your name on a candle and burn it, place the vellum with your enemy inscribed thereon and shove it to the back of the freezer, some will dose you with herbal tinctures or conjure you a talisman from the bones of long-dead tiny birds. And yes, I do all that, except the freezer trick. They are all deep and ancient techniques. We also sometimes do other things not meant for this book but that's neither here nor there. This form of healing is that of food and physical training. They also work. And while these arts are usually a matter of knowledge and body-to-body conversation, you have this grimoire. It is based solely and only on personal experience, so I promise there will be no parlor tricks, table-rapping or snake-oil.

This is your new health story but I'm beginning with the dark arts of how to banish a sleazebag because they exist. They are the tricksters in myth and indigenous lore. *Loki* in a mortal man's body. If you encounter one of these do not feed it. Do not stroke it, or its ego. Stare the beastie in the face, but carefully. You never know whether they will turn on you and hurt you. Even kill you. Because as we all know, witch or not, we are murdered all the time. Or betrayed. Or whatever abuse you hide away, because of shame or impotence. Because of the time you wept when you were raped. Verbally physically or psychically abused. Were smirked at or treated like an object. In a courtroom where some other sleazebag worked very hard to make you out to be a liar. We are mainly hurt because we are women. What is that? There is, after all, never another reason. To you nice blokes? Excellent. I have met one or two of you, through a martial art, our poetry, in fitness and healing, in my covens, across from me at my tarot table, in a show, for a secret conversation.

A BOOK OF SHADOWS/A GRIMOIRE

I am small and lean. I am a poet, a teacher, a medicine woman, a linguist and a warrior, and therefore I am mighty. If you choose to put the techniques from this manual—grimoire—into practice, the healing could also work for you. You will also become strong Does that mean you will never encounter *Loki*? Don't be fooled, for even a minute. Of course you will. You already have.

I'll explain. I recently upgraded my training practice because I wasn't hitting certain muscle groups, and today I'm getting on with the new program. After my warm-up I complete four sets of pull-ups, before heading to the Smith Machine for a weightless squat session. And then things go to shit.

Loki walks away from the squat rack, dragging his knuckles along the floor, wafting hypermasculinity by way of his deodorant. He carries a pair of dumbbells to the incline bench and lifts them in preparation for his first rep. I sort of just stand by the squat rack bewildered.

In gym etiquette I communicate with him, mouthing the words *You finished here?* Indicating the racked up weights. He nods and grunts. He's left 180 kilos of plates on the bar. I'm impressed but I again get his attention.

"Can you put your weights away please?"

He drops his dumbbells, grinds me to dust with a look, and swaggers over. When he's close enough to bite me he says, "You're a fucking pain in the arse, you know that?"

I'm confused at this, because there are signs all over this gym that say, CLUB RULES: REPLACE YOUR WEIGHTS AFTER USE.

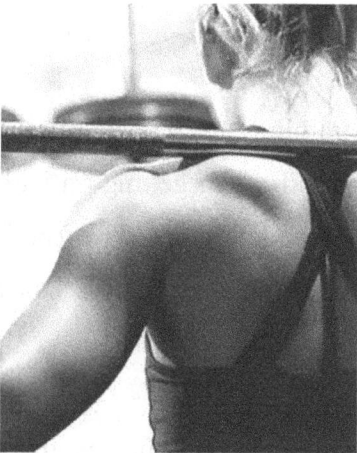

It takes me a few seconds to comprehend what's happening, and I smile at him, curious as to his looming outrage.

"Can you repeat that?" I ask. "I'm a bit deaf." And yes, it's a challenge. He's close enough to kiss me.

"You're a fucking pain in the arse." And he slowly, jerkily, removes the weight plates, body-language indignant. Now I'm angry.

You can kill him, you know. That seductive inner rat voice reminds me of all the years I trained in the martial arts. I hush it, but I've got my head tilted to one side and my hands on my hips. Making me appear bigger, I suppose, like the praying mantis, or a puffer fish.

"Just so I'm really sure, can you insult me one more time?" I say.

He wants to hit me, and I'm a nervous he might be on roids and that I just could have provoked a dangerous and unpredictable animal but, hey, what to do?

"*I said*—" He's communicating, somehow, through clenched teeth, and a razorblade-thin line of bloodless lips, "*You're a fucking pain in the arse, lady.*"

Lady?

(Must remember to let the manager know, in case I turn up dead in the side alley, for I am not done yet).) My curse on him is to remain unintimidated. He'll hate that. I'm supposed to say *sorry* and remove his toys for him.

I'm all woman, but I'm also androgynous. What does that mean?

Despite once having had copious quantities of fertile eggs, that were occasionally pierced by sperm resulting in offspring, I have always presented higher levels of testosterone than estrogen. I was still producing growth hormone—sufficiently to reach competition-level bodybuilding and run several martial art associations—in my forties, into my fifties and still today. Internally I have a uterus, externally I have pectoralis major and nipples, but no breasts. Not anymore.

Other than these two biological aspects, all else is uncertain. This is not uncommon, but others like me don't always realize what is happening. Why they behave differently to those of the seeming-same gender. Why they display an attitude not in accord with the social profiling of female or male.

Several years ago, post-menopause, I was advised by a medical expert that every woman has, or will "get", osteoporosis. Like other people get puppies or herpes. A given, simply because of gender.

ANDROGYNY

I was a *lovechild*—aka a bastard—born in December 1951, at a catholic hospital called Mater Misericordia for goodness sake, to a sixteen-year-old girlchild who did not name, then, the man who had shot his sperm into her and, therefore, really, should have been understood as responsible. How many girls and women do you know who think *Oh, I think I'll get pregnant so that someone can take the child and deny me access for the term of my natural life.* Hmm? A pair of strangers bought me as a christmas present for the kid they'd acquired the year before. As a child I was termed a tomboy, and strange by some people's standards. I read too much. By thirteen I was one of the first Goths on the streets of Sydney, in the cavernous dark of bohemian Kings Cross, listening to sixties rock and roll. I had severe acne and was conducting séances. The faux-mother was upset by both. If you've ever heard of Mosman, in Australia, you'll understand. Toffs, the lot.

The dermatologist ran blood tests for my outrageous zits. The return-diagnosis was one of an over-abundance of male hormone. Bad news for a girl. I was also moody and artistic. Religious in an inappropriate way. A talker to spirits. He prescribed barbiturates to subdue me. Those were still the years of extreme gender divide and where my budding *witchiness* was very much a hushed virulence, thought evil. Like me. Anyone who raged against their cage was shunned. Or institutionalized. Shame was a gender-biased weapon. A very christian, pompous weapon. If we dobbed in a rapist, we were made to feel shame. Same if we told how we got the bruises.

Shame was used by families and the church, by schools and psychiatry. And psychiatry was BIG. Hysteria was passé by now, no thanks to Freud, but because of him we apparently suffered penis-envy. Everything WRONG about us was because we were not male.

GOLD RUSH

Today the shaming is age. And shaming is a gold rush. Women, either cis or trans, are the new consumers because we're not allowed to *look* old. Industries are thrilled by our fear of rejection.

Simultaneously, advertising explains that it is advantageous to age faster, so that the *one-way-doors-to-the-coffin* that are geriatric institutions—now called retirement villages or aged-care facilities—and the funeral industry, bank the profits while we are still fit, so that our families do not carry the burden of our inevitable frailty and corpishness. Shame follows us. Turns us into consumers of our own ageing process.

A decade ago, one of my adult offspring suggested, snidely, that I grow old gracefully. I asked what that meant, and I wondered who they had become. We are to be silent, dependent, cover our looseness or our fatness with old lady garments. Lauded at 80, for still being pretty, wearing pink lipstick, flowers in our hair. Keeping a bag packed for the day of *the fall*, like we did for labor. While men the same age pretend to govern the world.

STYLE

I had my septum pierced a year later. Is that graceful enough?

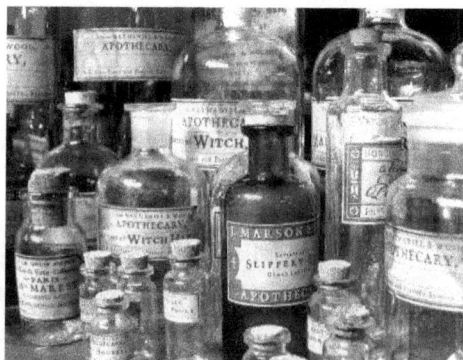

...

Way back in the days before the internet and the mobile phone I sat in the kitchen of a cold old stone cottage deep in the high country of Victoria, in the heart of a bitter winter, flabby with self-neglect, twenty-or-so kilograms over my current, natural body-weight, eating lemon spread and greasy lasagna when I was confronted by a photograph of Linda Hamilton, in the role of *Sarah Connor*, changing the clip on her fully-automatic weapon, in the full page article advertising *Terminator 2*, of a Saturday newspaper. I didn't know at the time how much that image would affect me.

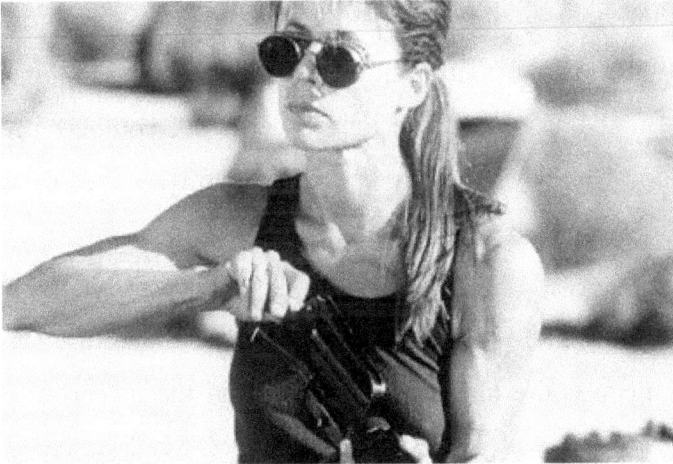

Image from the movie (Tristar)

This revised and expanded edition is for every gender but specifically women: every weird person, wildling and future soil. Everyone who understands that magic is not a stage trick. That doctors, yes, can save a life and set a bone, but some just fulfil what they can get away with, take the money for pushing the thalidomide.

Believing the hype. In all the years of training in Australia they also only learn about forty hours of nutrition, get a fifty percent pass, pass out the pill-du-jour and oh can, therefore, be snake oil merchants and quacks.

TRANSFORM OR DIE

A bleak and icy winter morning, the first of August 1991, and I woke before dawn aware, finally, of the play of my life: a tired, physically unmotivated thirty-nine-year-old psychic, witch and hoodoo woman. Author of two book, high priestess of a coven and mother of three living children. Knowing, despite the semblance of success and honesty, that I didn't like me much anymore. An unquiet soul. An unease growing more and more intense. An intuitive certainty that I wouldn't live long or well if I couldn't invoke my inner Sarah Connor. My body begging me to wise up. I didn't know how, so it was a matter of winging it.

The first thing I did was to radically alter eating. Raw greens and soup. Gone was the lasagna and bread, and the macaroni cheese. I was now relying completely on gut instinct. My kids hated me but that was not a deterrent. A person has to pull up from the rabbit hole down which we all freefall at some stage of life. Asthma was a recent ailment and, truth is, we can die. You, me, someone we care about. Sometimes younger than we intended or believed was destiny.

We can fuck up without insight or wise-woman-hoodoo. We really can. So let's not.

This changed eating regime promoted the need to move lots, so began the walking. Fast and striding. Down bush tracks. Rugged up in a thick old ex-army great-coat and woolly hat. Mittens and motor-bike boots to prevent freezing in that springtime of Victoria's high country, with its sleet and frost-biting winds.

Within the first week I was clocking up ten kilometers a day. Digestion and consciousness became calm. Thought more complex, a bit like a Rubik's cube adept. Excuses rejected.

EXCRETING EXCUSES

What was that? Not sure about anything, anymore, I deeply, sincerely, and suddenly realized what I didn't want. Now change becomes literal when a person learns that all the blood, and every cell in the human body, is in a constant process of birth and death and life:

> *The typical human being, for example, contains some 6,000 million million molecules of the protein haemoglobin in the blood. Every second 400 million million of these molecules are destroyed, but their concentration in the blood is unaffected because they are replaced as fast as they are removed.* ~~*The Death of Forever*, Darryl Reanney, Longman Cheshire, 91

Time to abandon a worn-out relationship, farewell friends, forego the responsibilities I had accumulated towards hundreds of people, my house and many of my possessions. I had a yard sale, and even gave away a hundred-year-old, full-length mink coat, gifted to me by an artist friend a few years previously. Who needs fur in the tropics? Because that was my destination.

My younger two kids, aged eight and nine, were loaded into the car alongside the dog, the cats, books, toys, clothes and a few necessities. I drove in my doubtful EH Holden station-wagon (with a goat-trailer towing whatever didn't breathe), towards the far north coast of New South Wales with Virginia, another woman of witchery, riding metaphorical *shotgun*, the children spread out over the back seat with five newborn kittens. Inside me was a bubble of excitement that needs neither explanation or justification.

Have you ever yearned for freshness and a chance to write a new chapter in your life? Have you ever felt like that? To rip out a page of two on how to behave, according to someone's idea of god, and burn them as fire-starters on the off-ramp. Some might say you are running away but you tell them *No, I'm running to*.

Arrival was October 1991. Just short of me turning forty.

BELIEVING IN YOURSELF

We moved onto Bunjalung country, on the outskirts of Byron Bay. An acre belonging to a student from my final tarot class. He'd said, *it's yours as long as you want, I'm staying down here however-long, reading tarot and surfing Bells Beach*. Home was a camper van, an annex and a large tent. Broken Head. Swampy bushland not far from town. The children began school and Virginia and I discovered the pleasure of anonymity, sunshine and a cappuccino at a sidewalk café. A quiet, alternative eco-environment where everyone smiled all the time.

We shed the skins of necessity that had belonged to the restrictive culture in which I had become enmeshed over the past several years and discovered the intense taste-sensations of food we hadn't even known existed. Salad without iceberg lettuce. With a rainbow of leafy greens, coconut, pippies, avocados, mango straight off the tree.

MARTIAL ART—THE ROOKIE

A couple of weeks passed before I saw a sign above the Old Norco building that said *Hapkido Association* (a Korean style of martial art), and I asked the kids if they wanted to give it a try.

I was spread-legged and dejected on the visitor bench at the rear of the dojo, that first night, watching the class. thinking *I can do that.*

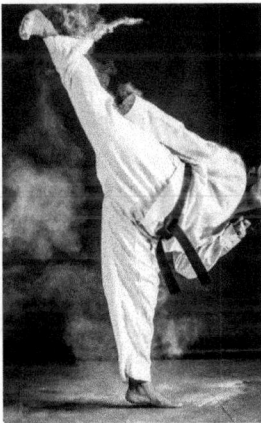

while the mantra of my internal rat voice nagged like a demented husband that I was way too old. Better just read tarot because I was also far too unstable emotionally, scared and unfit. So I began to heal from koyaanisqatsi. I started a daily routine of pleasure, passion and self-induced pain that became a technique (of several that life have been thrown at me) destined to strip away the illusions of a lifetime, a process still ongoing over two decades later. Magic, of course.

FOCUS AND CONCENTRATION

The martial art was complicated and exacting, in a straightforward and unassuming way. The discipline was a matter of ideal, and the integration of mind/body became a new focus. I progressed well, zooming through grading days with ease. But to kick the bag? To punch it? I had good form but no physical strength.

PERFECT THE FORM

Aruptananda became a close friend. A young gay man, a black-belt who was about my size, with the same birthday. We practiced moves and katas naked, or partially, on the soft sandy shores of Kings Beach. Training in leaps over incoming surf. Wrestling in oil. Bronzing (the Basel cell carcinomas came later). Him watching the young men go by, distracted. Me laughing.

In the dojo, however, it was a different matter...

> *Perfect the form,* he said. *Find your center. Feel the power within that center and let all of you be there. Send the unthought, perfect power out from there without force.*

Project the energy – the ki – calmly and deliberately. Perfect the form and the choreography will become second nature.

THE CENTER/THE DANTIANS

That center is two things: one, it's no-place at all that you can find except that you know it is there, and two, your body feels it in what's called the *dantian* (loosely translated as *elixir field,* or *sea of qi*) that, in martial arts, is the belly and genitals.

THE THREE TREASURES

The three *dantians* are collectively known as *the three treasures*: The central dantian, *jing,* is approximately two inches below the navel and is the source of energy that builds the physical body and allows us to develop and use *qi* and *shen*. Interesting now that we know that the intestine has a brain larger than that in our skulls, and that the microbiome is the ecology of health or disease.

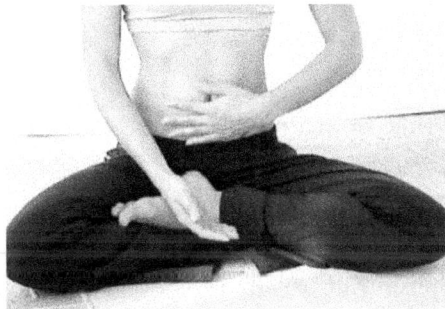

The medial dantian, *qi,* is around the heart, lung and stomach area. It is concerned with food and air. The head-height dantian, *shen,* is just higher than the eyebrows and is synonymous with consciousness. *Dantian* is often used interchangeably with the Japanese *hara* and the Chinese *fu*.

PUMPIN' IRON—THE ROOKIE

I began resistance training – working with free-weights – to enable progress at Hapkido. Only to discover that pumping iron was the perfect expression of the projection of power that my body, mind and spirit required (separate here for understanding's sake).

ME 'N' YOU

Responsibilities you have, probably through necessity, taken on in your life can be stored in your body, like an unmoving stasis. A heavy, metal, straight jacket around really being happy. That old deadness dwells in both cellular and muscular memory. The amount of weight you can pump can be the perfect balance, therefore release, of this stored, static corrosion. Oxidization. Weight training releases pressures trapped within one's physiology. A kind of *dirty ki*.

You can unlock this built-up repression, but to completely let go you'll want to release what you have unwittingly learned as, *hey, this is heavy!* It is relaxing to sweat and groan and have your eyes feel like they're popping out of their sockets. Like a hazy, autumn afternoon. Same as when a parking-spell works consistently. You simply need to know how firmly to hold your *dantian*, how strongly to hold your back, how rooted to the ground, the chair, the bench you've necessarily to be.

LEARNING TO BE STRONG

It's odd. I think it's odd. When people think of a healer—a medicine woman—they see a person that does not look like them. Someone with a bag of potions and a chant, with bells and crystals and perhaps rum, or incense, or bright shiny alien leaves. They don't see a body builder. They don't see a ragged pair of tracky-daks.

So, do you have to dress the part? Put feathers of dead birds in your hair and light candles when electricity could suffice? A nice lamp? Buy into the façade?

Healing though strength training happened at a local gym every morning, five days out of seven, after I'd seen the kids off to school. This was the witching hour. Training. The exploration of muscle and tendon, sinew, neural communication and mycelium/matrix network. There were practical transformations. Skills new to me as a healer. I accrued knowledge that had never occurred to me as anything but theoretical. I'd only mainly used herbs and spells all my adult life.

This mysterious inner landscape, in practicality, was as alien to both me and the alternative healing community as the mountains at the bottom of the ocean. Bodywork information came from textbooks; it was not experienced like this. Not ever before. After several months I became noticeably, and obviously physically different. My petite, lean frame had begun curving surprisingly on arm, back, shoulder, legs. These were muscles. I was altering my entire physiology with free weights and Hapkido.

A SPECTACULAR EDUCATION

I read articles in bodybuilding magazines. Observed and questioned the fitter of the athletes at the gym. To question everyone who seemed to know what they were doing. I watched their form, their favored exercises for certain muscle-groups. I discovered which exercises focused most accurately on an individual body part like distinct breeds of puppies at puppy-preschool. I learned how muscle grows through foods and adequate rest, what-not-to-do and specific needs and necessities, all of which I will pass on to you.

REFINEMENT—THE BEGINNING

Over the years I refined the techniques for both myself and my many students of widely varying genders, ages and fitness levels. I also now have a deep and honoring love-affair with food. All of us are living-earth, we share a secret about trust, but I'll tell you about that later when we gather in the kitchen, by the fire and the cauldron, sharing spit-roasted, slow-cooked goat, and stories of the long-ago when we were wolves and ravens and bears, before we lost the hunt and the forage, and the ancient trackways through the forest of our ancestors.

...

'THERE IS NO BEAUTY
WITHOUT SOME

STRANGENESS.'

[POE]

MEDICINE WOMAN SURVIVE AND THRIVE—
RAZOR DAYS

It's been a process taking years, like butchering a mammoth on the kitchen bench, with a blunted and rusted cutthroat razor that a potential grandfather once stropped, the dismissal of affection, the branches of this living tree:

You, for your casual *Darlings* that dissolve into weeks, then months, because you are distracted by your jazz or whatever, until I can turn my back on your empty how are you and place you in one of the plethora of Canopic jars that I have within this edifice that I call me.

Me, slipper satin and ornate brass astrolabes, tattooed ears, huge round tables lacquered in flawless Chinese red, lipsticks of every hue except plum—I despise the color plum except on plums—theatre curtains in midnight blue hiding the pantomime of my childhood, and books that reach the lofty, glass-domed widows' walk high above me. And you: those of you who haven't fled or been stuffed within the jar.

You, for the panic when I suggest I might need a room if things go weird. You, for over-thinking the past and casting me as the enemy while still professing love. The others, one by one.

This is not about being perfect, no, it's because I am tired of trying to be.

You, for never laughing even though you smile. I understand your desperation but I am not your psychiatrist, or your mother.

Others hang from these gnarled boughs, fruit fresh to rotting and more will fall.

Initiating conversation one too many times.

Life still has this woman's name. This woman's mind. And it is confounded by body language that says most things, stutters and pauses that say most else, and that *undoneness* that comes out of the mouth trying in vain to justify through distraction or remission as though I am blind or cattle.

Few remain with bright plumage to my eyes.

It's not that I want to carve the beast or sever the limbs with the all-but-bladeless razor; I so desperately don't. However...

Rather than hold it to my own throat I will use it to sever the fruit from the limb and butcher the mammoth in my kitchen until I am soil.

...

The worst thing about
being lied to is
knowing you weren t
worth the truth.

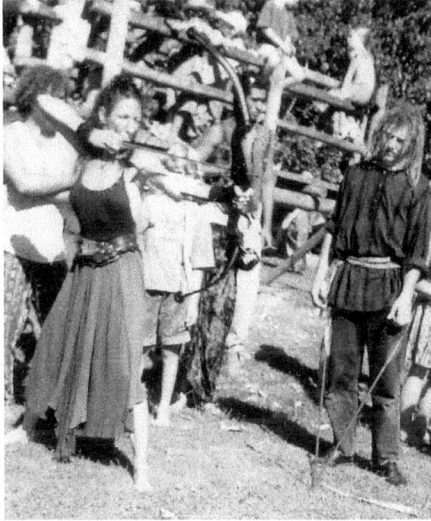

Ly (with bow). Before PPD poisoning

Exercise: is the exercise for the specific muscle group.

Sets: are the numbers of times you'll repeat the same exercise.

Reps: are the numbers of repetitions of a movement within a set.

On Living: there doesn't have to be a reason.

PLEASE MEMORIZE

. . .

Dear Diary,

My belly, my breasts, my bum, my face

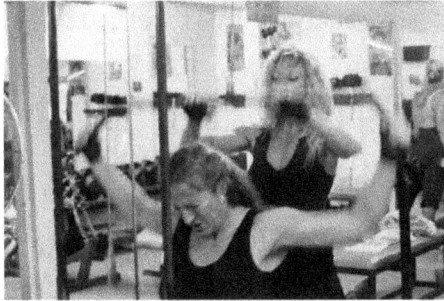

Cate and Ly, Byron Gym, Old Norco Building, 1994

Everything here is based on experience. Some of the technical terminology has been 'information-learned' but that is always of little or no relevance if not understood through real-life doing.

Bodybuilding is also called resistance training and weight training. It can also be body-shaping or body-toning, if you train lightly. An easy body/mind-enhancing technique. The terminology is based on a complete (so far) understanding of synergy of body, mind and spirit integration.

GRUNT

I have mainly worked with women and I am assured of one thing – most of us are afraid of our bodies. We often belittle our significance in the world, and our capacity for prowess and excellence. If it's not done to us we do it to ourselves. What *is* that? We also possess an unfounded fear of self-harm based on a deep and confused lack of trust and adequate information. The lack of clearly marked trackway to well-informed sources.

Many are too embarrassed to power out a breath, let alone grunt, pant or groan through the final repetition necessary to create transition, so we initially tend to underplay the weight. I wonder, sometimes, if the whole problem hasn't arisen from an antique, albeit deep-rooted denial of self-expression. And yes, when we do an exercise cleanly we sound like we are orgasming.

SPELLCASTING

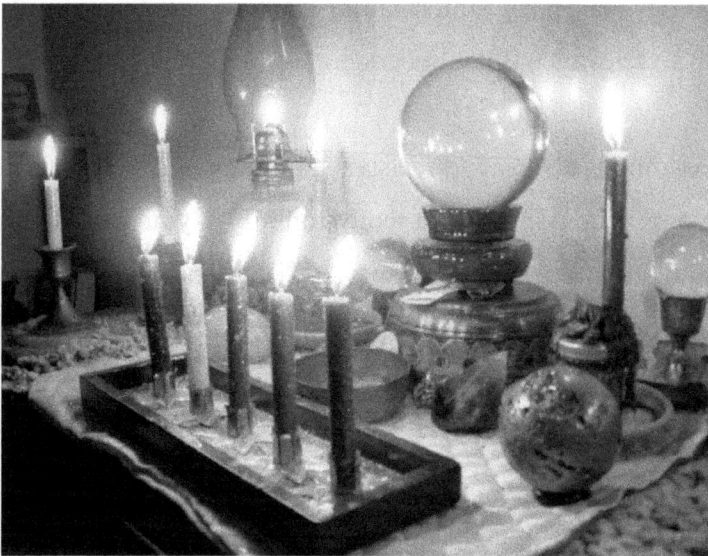

Some have a rootless fear of becoming like competition bodybuilders. But that'll never happen unless we want it. Outcomes to healing will depend as much on *genetics* as on determination, and inherent body-type will come into play as you shed excess body fat.

To arrive at competition-level bodybuilding or body-shaping would take you hours, days, years of absolute dedication. It is also common knowledge that many competition-level bodybuilders use anabolic steroids. Other than having chosen not to, I have no opinion on this.

Medical research has done little to no serious enquiry into the effects of anabolic steroids on long-term or overall health and until they do I refuse judgment, remembering that anything excessive is potentially harmful.

So, your first spell is the elimination of fear, while taking care and responsibility. It might assist you, about now, to work some candle magic, or make a poppet of yourself in the image of your inner warrior.

EXCESS BODY FAT

The quantity and *quality* of body fat that anyone stores will have a deciding influence on our appearance when we are healing from whatever trauma caused us to consume home-brand pizza and ice cream. We want brown fat but not white fat. As Dr. Pam Peeke[3] explains:

White fat has many purposes. It provides the largest energy reserve in the body. It's a thermal insulator and cushion for our internal organs, and cushions during external interactions with our environ-

---

[3] https://www.womenshealthmag.com/health/a19896462/fat-facts

ment (that's code for a soft landing when we fall on our bum!). It is a major endocrine organ, producing one form of estrogen as well as leptin, a hormone that helps regulate appetite and hunger. It's also got receptors for insulin, growth hormone, adrenaline, and cortisol (stress hormone). So, it's a myth that fat cells just sit there and do nothing all day long!

Excess body fat is shed through the eating magic that we will turn to later, and via your outward breath during cardio-vascular workouts. The good thing about body fat is that it will provide you with a head start on the thin person. If you have stored fats, they will actually help you get stronger faster. Always there is more than one reason, especially in women, for obesity, and, be sure, even some very lean women retain body fat when their metabolism is super-fast.

CANNIBALISM AND INSIGHT
Our bodies, when threatened by inadequate supplies of nourishment (insulin) will cannibalize our own muscle (catabolism) before resorting to life-sustaining fat.

The dilemma of personal physical comfort is an individual thing, and several factors come into play. It is your choice to explore which of these are relevant to you.

Excess fats in the diet = excess fats stored within the body *overall*. Simple sugars (monocarbohydrates, including fructose. And, be sure, these products are in many, if not all, pre-packaged, processed and refined foods) will settle around the thighs, hips, belly and bum. People who consume copious quantities of booze look ten months pregnant, with thin legs and arms causing a deformed appearance. Why? Alcohol is made up of high quantities of simple sugars. The liver spends so much time processing the alcohol that inadequate metabolism results. Yeast-based beverages can trigger candida, or thrush, in a prevalent body, especially when put together with monocarbohydrates. Simple sugars are a time-bomb for the pancreas, preventing the regulation of natural insulin levels and often leading to Type 2 diabetes.

Estrogen-dominance will also cause bloating, fluid retention and a tendency to store fats. Get rid of plastic, and if you do happen to have a plastic drinking bottle (please recycle it and use stainless steel or reinforced glass) don't ever leave it in the daylight, sunlight or anywhere hot as plastic is a petrochemical derivative and is almost solely responsible for the world-wide phytoestrogen epidemic. And phthalates are dreadful (more on that later).

Too many hours between meals and eating large quantities of food at a sitting also inhibits metabolism, as can a lack of essential hydrochloric acid in the stomach, preventing sufficient breakdown in the digestive function and leading to excess storage of waste in the intestine. Nourishment is lost this way, because nutrients are distributed throughout the body through the walls of the large intestine. Fruit, for example, just kind of slides past the stomach and into the gut where its properties are assimilated. That's why you often feel hungry if simply consuming fruit. Fruit, however, is a big story that I'll also get to.

FREE WEIGHTS AND SHEDDING EXCESS BODY FAT

When there is an excess (repeat: *excess*) of body fat you work with lighter weights and higher repetitions than someone with an already lean physique as this allows the muscles to tone, and your inner greyhound to trust you. Foods that induce fat storage, in environments that are not cold all the time, are always the result of a lack of information or from being stressed by circumstances and needing to self-protect. Don't expect to achieve a lean body based on other forms of exercise. You are building muscle which is heavier than fat. Take care to maintain a healthy objectivity and avoid weighing yourself.

When there is little or no *excess* body fat, a standard 8 to 12 repetition set is where the beginner gets the greatest gains.

Understand that the *lower the reps* and *the higher the weight* then the *more the muscle-mass*, provided you get ample protein. Do, at the most, 12 repetitions of an exercise unless you're toning or shaping, then 15 to 20 reps are preferred.

TRAIN TO HEAL

Train to heal three or four exercises per body-part, two body-parts per workout day (except abs) until you know your magic and the web of communication with yourself is established and clear. Later, after about four to six months, you will increase your weights as a matter of course. Until you plateau. You're an animal. A puppy or a pony. You've learned the laziest way to get what you want. When this inevitably happens, experiment with heavier weights and less reps in what are called *straight sets*. Or in pyramiding sets. Or strip sets (I'll go into terminology later but for now let's just get the gist of the process). Or you'll want to super-set, or even play around for a week or two, just to break predictable patterns. Familiarize yourself with the chapter on MUSCLE GROUPS. It is inevitable that, should you continue resistance training for healing, you will come to utilize all the techniques, as well as explore many more.

THE HEALING DIARY

Over the first few weeks/months write up a diary documenting

- The food and drink you consume

- The program that you are currently implementing

- The quantity of weight and when you up it

- The addition of new techniques

- Emotional changes, life changes, witchy realizations and magical moments

- The things you forgot you knew

- How much you like being you. If not, why not?

...

THE
WORDS
YOU
SPEAK
BECOME
THE
HOUSE
YOU
LIVE IN

Dear Diary,

In my head there's a rat voice telling me I can't...

Hydration

Endorphins

Form

Breathing

Mind/body linkage

Focus

Recovery

Not necessarily separately or in this order

Food (nutrition: both the eaten and the emotional)

Supplementation

Relaxation

The body: proteins and sugars

And just a little more personalization before we get technical

...

ON THE EXECUTION OF AN EXERCISE

Supposing you're clear of fear and you say *I'm going for it,* and you power out those reps as hard and as fast as you can. I'm going to observe you for a few minutes, knowing from your body-communication that you're just starting out, before I worry whether to say anything or just shut up. Because you're jerking. Harming yourself and also getting into a dangerous habit.

I'm likely to say something, to explain that you're missing the muscle. You will get pumped, sure, but you might as well go join the circuit class for all the muscularity you'll be developing, let alone strength. Plus, you'll probably end up stressing your joints to pieces and will spend months in physiotherapy. What will we call that: *un-healing*? Explore your boundaries and transcend them. You are a horse that's encouraged through the patience and expertise of the Whisperer. A whisperer who earns the faith and companionship of that horse.

ON RECOVERY

Taking days off training can be uncomfortable. You become almost addicted to endorphins, but you grow when you rest. Know that, where weights are concerned, you rip the fascia that encapsulates muscle when you train hard (it's chrysalis time) and the correct food and adequate rest, when you're *not* working out, fills the rips with new cells.

That's the healing.

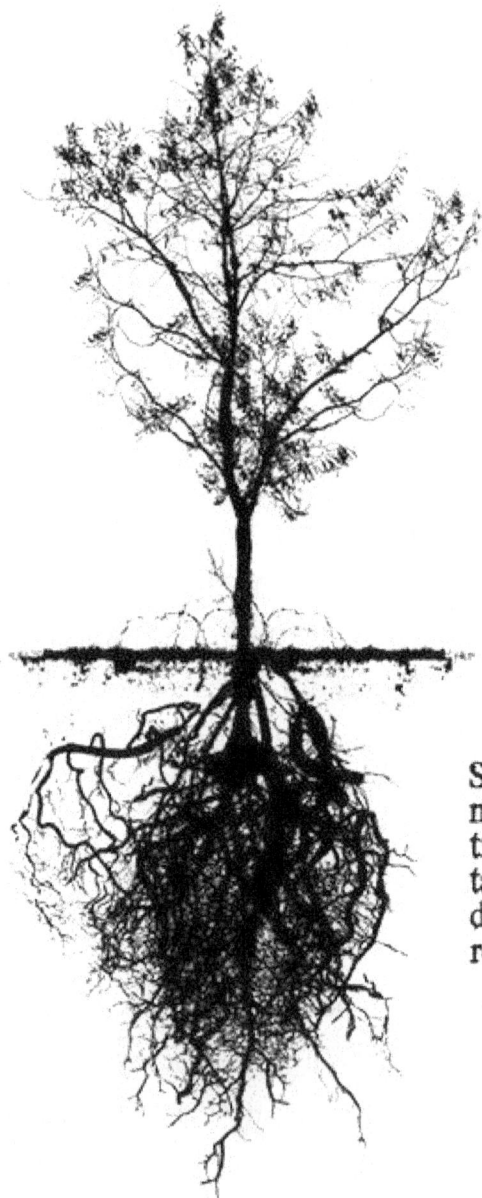

Storms
make
trees
take
deeper
roots.

...

Lies, like advertising, are paper cuts slicing, hardly recognized, into the minds of the gullible that want so desperately to acceptable. It is persuasive through its intended inexactness, its very vagueness and cheery promise. I really don't understand the gain. I really, really don't understand what has been achieved, unless—Is it captivity? That would make more sense than all else.

Captivity.

The deliberate, devious, crushing, annihilation of the right to choose to be at odds with the captors.

I see it— "We have your soul, now. We have marked you. We have registered you somewhere. You are accountable. To us. We have your soul, in writing. You have agreed to this, or else your parents before you and those before them."

How did this happen? Why your parents before you, and those before them? How else can they live with the lie that they are satisfied unless they tell you that they are and become, therefore, justified in the continuance of the repetition of captivity.

"We have your soul. We have taken it from you by holding your existence to ransom against the possibility of being cast out. Don't forget, for a minute, what you could lose."

I really love you Mother. I really understand what you have hidden for millennia. Kept it as safe as you could. Protect the child. At all costs, protect the child. Protect it from its father who believes in the rod; who believes in his omnipotence; who thinks (because he's told) that he, and he alone, was made in the likeness of a 'god'. You haven't been able to, though, have you, Mother?

Maybe not.

But before you die, over and over again, into some far-flung future, with unshed tears of disillusionment hidden from those who would be harmed by your admission, by your possible co-operation, by your imagined guilt at having felt you'd been so obscene, or never good enough, to the mind of your husband or your master or your lord; or your sons—to the betrayal of your daughters. Hear me.

Some of us have escaped.

Keep the faith in forever, Mother, keep the faith. The treasure of your children—freedom—is occulted, for now. Rest certain. This too will pass for she will give them ice and she will make them run and you will have been warned for your instinct remains keen for you are not complacent. You are merely silenced.

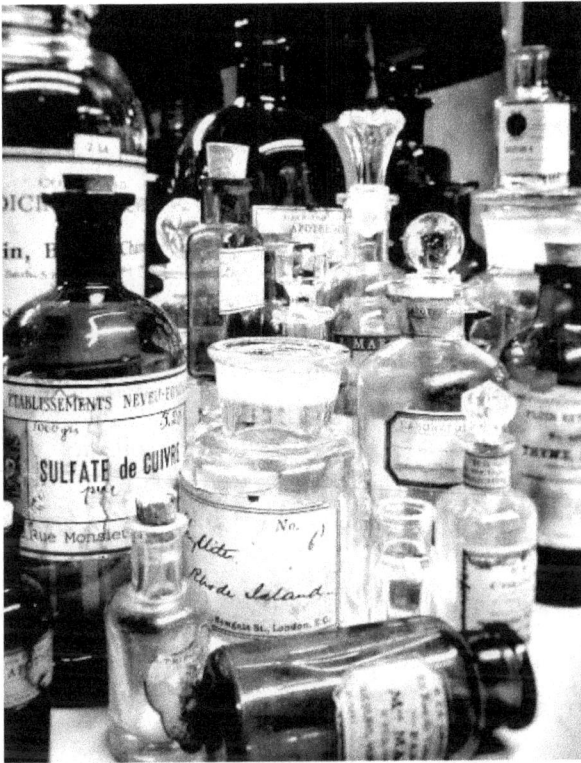

ENDOCRINE DISRUPTORS—VILE STUFF

We are exposed to endocrine disruptors through food and beverages consumed, pesticides applied, and cosmetics used. In essence, our contact with these chemicals may occur through diet, air, skin, and water.

Even low doses of endocrine-disrupting chemicals are unsafe. Our normal endocrine functioning involves very small changes in hormone levels, yet even these small changes can cause significant developmental and biological effects. This observation leads scientists to think that endocrine-disrupting chemical exposures, even at low amounts, can alter the body's sensitive systems and lead to health problems. And they are sperm killers, but that's another story.

BPA's

Bisphenol A (BPA) — used to make polycarbonate plastics and epoxy resins, which are found in many plastic products including food storage containers

Dioxins — produced as a byproduct in herbicide production and paper bleaching, are released into the environment during waste burning and wildfires

Perchlorate — a by-product of aerospace, weapon, and pharmaceutical industries is found in drinking water and fireworks

Perfluoroalkyl and *Polyfluoroalkyl* Substances (PFAS) — used widely in industrial applications, such as firefighting foams and non-stick pan, paper, and textile coatings

Phthalates — used to make plastics more flexible, they also hide in many forms of food packaging, cosmetics, children's toys, and medical devices

Phytoestrogens — naturally occurring substances in plants that have hormone-like activity, such as genistein and daidzein that are in soy products, like tofu or soy milk

Polybrominated diphenyl ethers (PBDE) — used to make flame retardants for household products such as furniture foam and carpets

Polychlorinated biphenyls (PCB) — included in the making of electrical equipment like transformers, and in hydraulic fluids, heat transfer fluids, lubricants, and plasticizers

Triclosan — found in some anti-microbial and personal care products, like liquid body wash

Oh, and interesting food for thought is that two of my friends are front line medical practitioners. They both, coincidentally, had tests for liver function not long into the *covid* epidemic. They both showed high degrees of disorder. Turns out it was from the alcohol content in hand sanitizers.

ON BREATHING

Strength training and maintenance = Bodybuilding, sculpting, shaping, power—resistance training. A healing art. As far as I am aware, never written of, as such, by other healers, or those working the way of witch or medicine woman. Why not? It amazes me, as every *Eastern*[4] way of learning involves a physical discipline. Consider the Taoist saying: *The pen and the sword in accord.* So—

When considering breath, it's interesting to seek the philosophical origins in *Western* knowledge: *pneuma* is "air in motion, breath, wind." This is equivalent in the material monism of Anaximenes, as the element from which all others originate. It is *anima*, in Latin, and was originally used to describe ideas such as breath, soul, spirit or vital force. Jung began using the term in the early 1920s to describe

---

[4] I dislike the segregationist terminology of East and West but add it here for the sake of clarity and understanding

"the inner feminine side" of men (an outmoded ideology, implying behavior implicit to gender. I do not concede this). Here we are again, with a word dividing us into dualisms, adopted by psychology as a truism. A sad forgetting that we are all really breathing stratosphere; that the oxygen we inhale has always been here. Our ancestors and all our stories.

Anaerobically is how we train in this healing art (see Glossary). It's not soft, it's caught, used to flood muscle and blood, and surrenderred back out to the universe on exhalation. When you push, or pull, or lift, you've got to breathe. And not just inhale/exhale but *breathe. On* the exertion.

A student once commented, *my breathing is always so shallow*. Like that was it. End of conversation. I didn't talk about it with her right then because I was in the middle of my set and we don't chat when we're concentrating on what we're doing, or we can hurt ourselves, not heal. She'd already written this chapter into her grimoire, but she'd forgotten (everyone always does until it becomes second nature). Breathe in, hold, then crash the air out on the lift, push or pull. This is what the body does naturally in strenuous situations.

Deep breathing stimulates every part of you. Some people, when they begin, and exert themselves, experience a *rush*, become heady and almost faint. That's your brain taking in more oxygen. Others vomit. What you are doing is breathing sky.

You need to take a deep and meaningful inward breath. Be present. Suck it in, sharp and voluminous. Then pull it up from your *dantian* and push it out right at the toughest part of the execution of the exercise. By the time you reach your twelfth rep you'll be gritting your teeth and looking beautiful, and you'll sound like you're having an orgasm. You'll be the only one to know if you're faking, and wouldn't that be a waste when, if you added just two more plates to the bar, it would be the real thing?

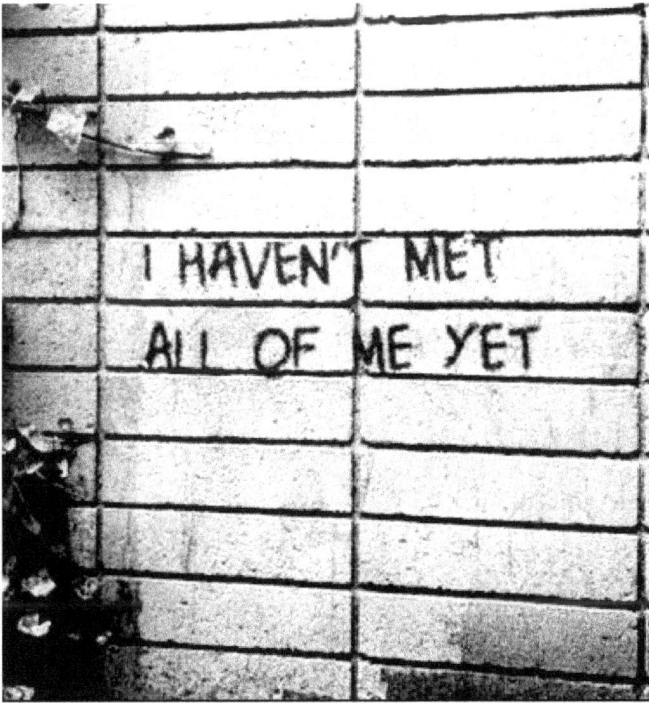

FAKE IT TILL YOU MAKE IT

Some women I've worked with have faked it (and I suppose they've got their reasons) but unfortunately they don't stay the distance required for healing. Life gets in the way. They are too sad, too scared, too tired. It all becomes too much of an effort. Unfortunately, they're often the ones to tell me what they expect their co-dependent partner to do to make them happy (like they couldn't just be happy for themselves). For the others who just can't hack it? Well, it's not for everyone. People who don't fake it, however, get to experience the *buzz*.

THE BUZZ (ENDORPHINS)

This kind of strength healing, when practiced consistently, releases chemicals (naturally-produced opiate-like relaxants): endorphins and endocannabinoids. These little bliss-balls get you high. They're responsible for you feeling fabulous after a workout, and not fatigued (that comes later in the day), as you wobble down a staircase (leg day), or quiver when you pick up your water-glass to wash down your highest quality, branched-chain amino acid supplement (any upper body part). The wobbles and the shakes, in legs and arms respectively, don't last more than a few weeks. Problematic, though, if you're a brain surgeon or a tattooist.

When you are stronger, and you as an animal have adjusted, you'll come out of the gym simply feeling pumped and mighty.

SIZE IS RELATIVE

Maybe not today (although I haven't tried it for a couple of years) but, last time I was asked I was able to lift the front of a small car out of a bog and could heave a bag of horse manure over my shoulder for the veggie garden. Size is a relative concept, and often people larger than you, sometimes younger than you, are vulnerable and fragile. Once my current GP had assessed that I was not a candidate for osteoporosis they confided in me that one woman under their care broke the metacarpal bones in her hand simply by opening a car door. That's the silent harm that not learning this form of healing will cause.

I admit I did the same once. But on a punching bag. The day I bought it. I was too enthusiastic and did not take the time to apply my wraps. Endorphins (already mentioned) are such strange small friends that I felt no pain until the following day. But broke the little bones in my hand? Yes. Happily, (is that even appropriate?) not due to osteoporosis, despite being at least forty-five summers alive by then. Just negligence and a delusion of invincibility.

THE POWER OF WATER

You're hard into your workout and you get a cramp. Drink some water. Before you train drink water. When you're hot, drink water. Dehydration will take from you what you have striven so hard to achieve. We are waking, and healing, skeletal muscle. She needs both water and glycogen to function properly, as well as adequate potassium and magnesium.

Dehydration is not simply obvious when you're thirsty (and I drink about two liters during a session). Your skin will also improve. If you are exerting yourself and you forget to hydrate, it may be too late. It's even better if the drink you have with you when you train contains electrolytes as these replace depleted cell salts. Be aware, however, that commercial brands can be costly, and you will definitely want to avoid the ones with simple sugars in them, especially aspartame and any GMO sugars like corn syrup.

On a trip around the world in 2003 I was in Switzerland for a week. Zurich. One of the people in the apartment where I stayed was violently ill with kidney pain. This was the summer that the first unprecedented heatwave crippled Europe. Approximately 11,000 people died. The thing was, the people I spoke to had no idea that drinking water would heal them. In Australia hydration is a matter of common knowledge. Summers here are always hot. The man with the kidney agony took three days to urinate out the crystals that heat sickness had caused. The point is to understand your physical needs and to not rely on tradition or habit to expect to cope.

HEAL OR HARM – ON SELF SABOTAGE

You can cannibalize yourself: *catabolism*. You can eat your own muscle from the inside. If you do not fuel yourself adequately you will become weaker, debilitated, open to disease. You lessen your immune system's defenses and you will suffer irritability, anxiety and exhaustion.

INSULIN AND THE INSULIN SPIKE

After a heavy training session your body requires *some* form of sugar to trigger insulin. Many protein powders and workout drinks, however, are chockablock with detrimental simple sugars. *Encarta's Interactive Encyclopedia* defines insulin as "a pancreatic hormone that regulates the metabolism of carbohydrates and fats by controlling blood glucose levels." Insulin is necessary for building muscle and to transports nutrients to the organs in the body. This includes muscle cells and fat cells.

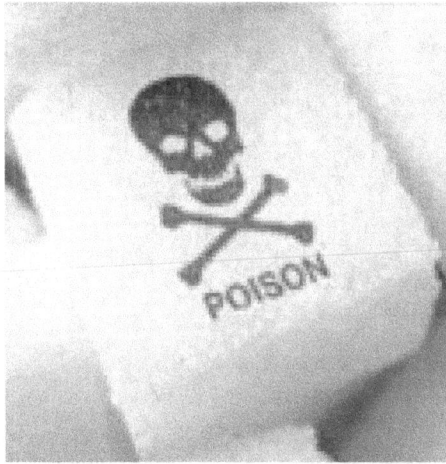

While insulin is driving amino acids and glucose into muscle cells, it also prevents the leaking out of these nutrients from the muscle cells that usually occur in response to training or illness.

Insulin aids each cell to volumize. Its effect is anabolic. Bodywork demands it. To increase stamina and improve endurance. It is important to realize insulin is used to increase muscle bulk because it stimulates the formation of glycogen which feeds your muscle cells during a workout.

Rather than suck on a protein shake during training, however, I will always eat a high fat, high protein meal, however small, half an hour to an hour before getting in my car, preferring to utilize that for energy rather than risk the long-term effects of loading up with sugars.

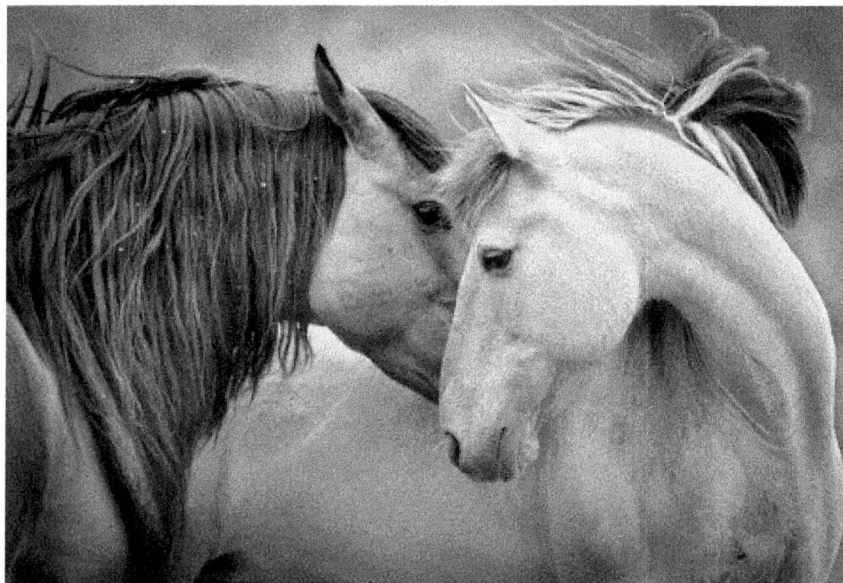

I take a few blueberries (chock full of antioxidants, fructose, vitamin C, manganese and potassium) with me. No fruit *juice*, however, as whereas glucose is evenly distributed throughout your body, fructose goes straight to the liver. All kinds of trouble there, re fatty liver. I consume this immediately after training. This will sustain me for the drive home and I will drop a scoop of high protein powder, a hit of B.C.A.A.'s (branch chain amino acids) in water, and blend them, once I'm in the door. Within twenty minutes of training. Only after this do I eat.

It's a simple fact that solid food can take hours to digest. You need energy beforehand.

Eat what will nourish you and not simply fill you: proteins, certain complex carbohydrates and specific fats. You are *not* going to under-train because that makes all this regenerative work pointless.

You're also not going to over-train because your muscles will devour themselves and you'll exhaust, leaving you susceptible to external pollutants. It is easier for your cells to gain needed energy, quickly, from muscle, when your body senses threat, rather than from stored fats. Unless you are in ketosis. It's a little like parenting correctly or being kind to animals. When you live with a horse and your witchery is the skill of a *whispe*rer, you would automatically want to train her with humor, kindness and honor. Horses, hounds and hunting hawks don't mind the pace when they know they can trust you, but you a) don't want to break their bodies and b) you *will not* break their spirits. Treat yourself likewise.

Over the coming months you will discover what your perceived limits were and, trust me, you will render them the illusions they have been. Execute perfect form for each exercise (if you're practicing what are known as cheats then do so with intent), use a spotter (that's someone who'll assist you with those last one or two reps) if possible, and work with a buddy if you can find someone you know and admire, someone who can match your incentive, keeping in mind that a partner should be someone sufficiently knowledgeable.

Use your intelligence to engage synergistically, with the muscles. Ligaments, tendons, breath, joints, bones and don't underthink the exercise.

Once you've established communication with yourself you will know honest intimacy, and it will be easier to do so again and again. This is where you'll gain super-cool benefits.

IS THAT A GUN IN YOUR POCKET OR ARE YOU JUST HAPPY TO SEE ME?

When can you expect to feel differently about who you are since you started? From day one. With the familiarity of techniques, you will have altered, utterly, however imperceptibly, in one month.

Muscles will begin to emerge from their compressed, cocooned, unappreciated little cave in your life, like a bear in the spring after a frozen winter hibernation.

You will have the pleasure of running your hand over your arm or your leg and letting escape a little *ooo* in about six months. A year later the *ooo* will become *ahhh!* By the time you have trained for between two and three years you'll be analytical, and instead of the *ahhh* you'll be: *these posterior delts needs more attention.*

But it never becomes boring. Even now, as an elder femme, I enjoy the shapes that muscle creates in movement. It is so easy to contemplate being an ecosystem—an environment.

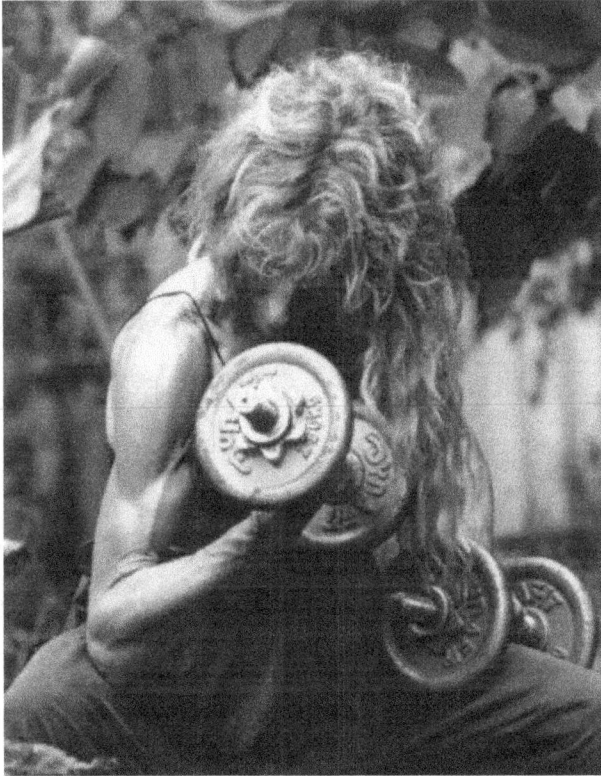

Ly at 42 summer, Byron Bay

After two years you're no longer flushed each time you greet someone who hasn't seen you since the before photo and who says, *what happened to you?* You are healed. You have treated the whole of you. You are literally a different creature.

You empathize with the power of animals and plants. Their nature will be understood. Their roots, their resilience will be *family*. With animals you'll admire with their lying about. You will have stopped believing that you are separate, somehow, from earth and you will no longer suffer the illness of delusion and loneliness. Think of the bacteria, that makes up so much of us, as living in a bright and healthy coral reef.

But, when you've traveled that far you will need to take special care not to let your training take over your life. Because it can.

LOSING DELUSION—THE HEALING DEEPENS

As you live and learn this healing art you'll realize all the *other* illusions of inadequacy that you accepted. You'll be the progenitor of change. Your resilience, the stress, will be proportionate to the experience. You'll not need to imagine yourself as other than you are. Fear is simply relative to experience. You'll need it—the adrenalin—to outrun that random pride of starving lions (or the equivalent) whose path you crossed by fate or bewitchment.

It's all so very mystical, magical and hoodoo.

...

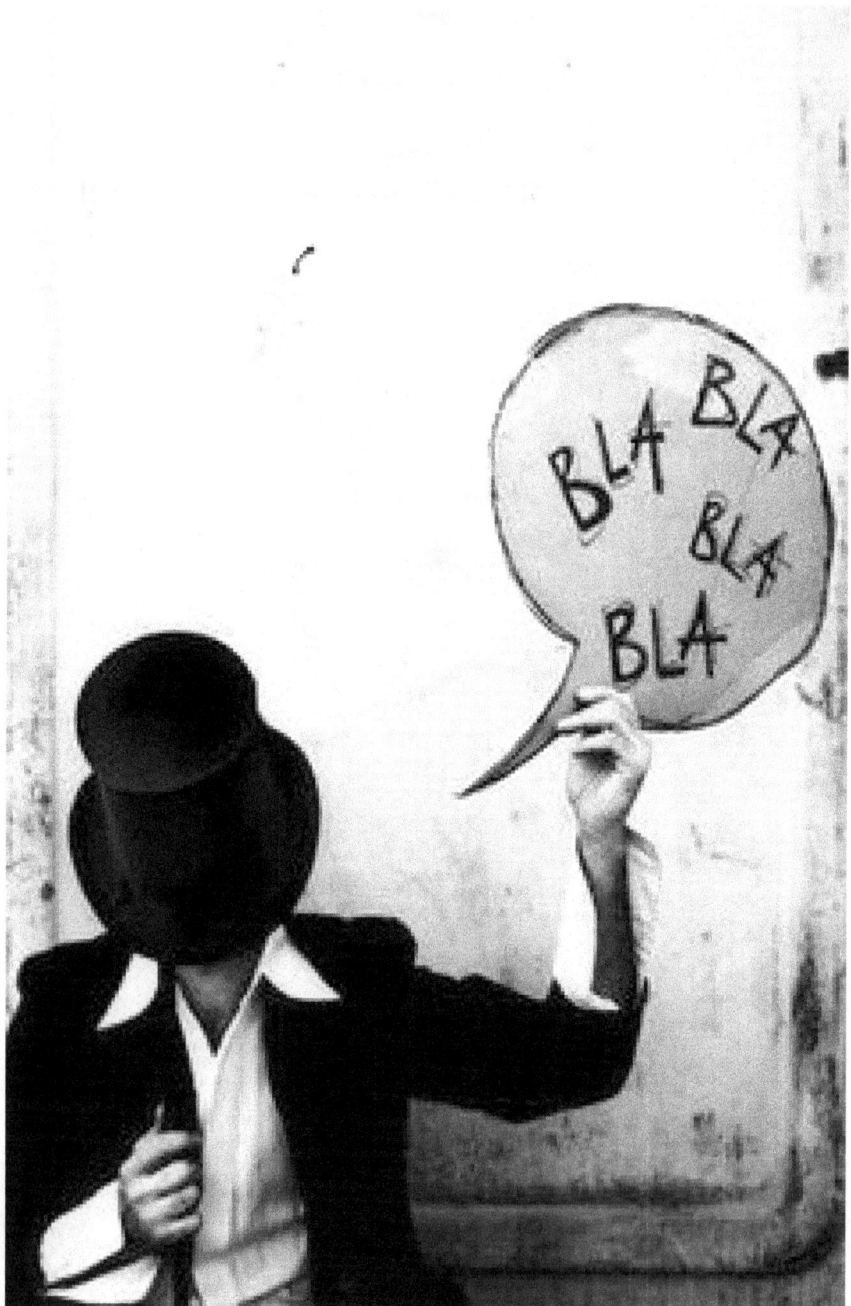

Sometimes I despise my ambition
because it constantly interferes,
because it demands I pay it attention,
because it constantly tells me how important it is

Sometimes I despise my pride.
If it would stop annoying
me the way it does at least once a day
I could live in affluent squalor
with stuff I collect or steal or beg.

Darlings,

you don't pay rent

in a tent.

...

TO DIET OR NOT TO DIET

A misnomer of a word, lovelies. There is no such thing as a diet in the general and commercial sense. Diet is neither losing nor gaining weight. Diet comes from the Greek word *DIAITA* which means a way of living and is defined by the dictionary as the daily fare and food, about its nutritive value or its effects on you.

The word nutrition is *the act or process of taking nourishment; especially the process by which food is assimilated and converted into tissue in living organisms.*

By eating inadequately, you are stifling, suppressing, restricting, and even destroying your natural regenerative capabilities. One can eat – and eat lots – and die of malnutrition.

If you become fixated, or obsessive in your attitudes to food, and subsequently extoll to others that: *it is wrong to eat this or that. Wrong* is such a rubbish word, isn't it? Just another interfering binary. What matters is *knowledge* woven from researched and trustworthy information, keen self-awareness and sensitivity. And common sense. None alone of these qualities is sufficient, however. If you have the former and you develop, or rather let loose, your animal nature, you will unleash the latter.

Other species will instinctively avoid substances that are dangerous.

Or suffer the consequences. Let an animal spend too much time under the influence of certain dysfunctional human eaters, however, and you'll have them craving chocolate, cheese, cake, chips and ice-cream. Why? Because people introduce these things to our cousins. Even though, as a result, this will undoubtedly cause disease, and shorten their life span.

tomorrow

(noun)

a mystical land where 99% of all human productivity, motivation and achievement is stored

Dear Diary,

Coercive control has affected my life by…

I live with a form of synesthesia. I see words, whether spoken or written. I see them literally. This is an extension of being psychic and *seeing* a client experiencing life. So when people throw words away without realizing what they are saying it either hurts in a very visceral way or surprises. My point...

She's unraveling.
That'll be your undoing.
She's falling to pieces.
She's coming unstuck.
She can't keep it together anymore.
She needs to get over herself.

Then—

She's holding up pretty well all things considered.
She comes up alright with a bit of spit and polish.
She's just killing time.
Mutton dressed up as lamb.

She has to meet the deadline.

What I can't see is the expression *unfuckable*. It does not engender an appropriate image.

Dear Diary,

This week ...

I stopped resistance training, as a discipline and healing art, in my early fifties, to fully concentrate on Aikido and Iaido. Then, within a few years, through circumstances and betrayal but the men in these clubs, I washed my hands of both of them. I slowly, and inexplicably, gained ten kilos. My body-weight prior to then had been around fifty-two kilos and I did not understand what was happening. Not fully. I was through the sweats and brainlessness of menopause but other problems: mood swings, exhaustion, insomnia and anxiety dogged me. Low self-esteem. And depression. I knew about all the rest but depression? Not always from sadness.

HEAVY METALS. CURSE AND CURE

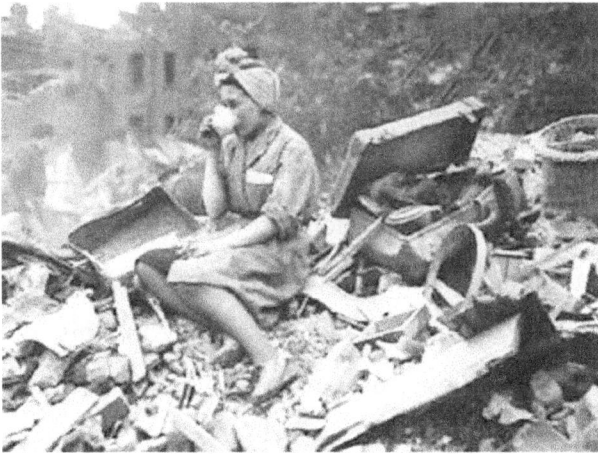

I stopped resistance training, as a discipline and healing art, in my early fifties, to fully concentrate on Aikido and Iaido. Then, within a few years, through circumstances and betrayal but the men in these clubs, I washed my hands of both of them. I slowly, and inexplicably, gained ten kilos. My body-weight prior to then had been around fifty-two kilos and I did not understand what was happening.

The *depression* was caused by mercury poisoning. Dawson Warren, my local doctor, savvy to my usual perennial healthiness had me tested for heavy metal poisoning. When the blood results returned dangerously elevated levels of the neurotoxin, Dawson prescribed an antidepressant for the debilitating moods, but also massive doses of vitamin C, B12, psyllium husk, and a product called Vital Greens. I was to dump my exorbitantly expensive bottle of Omega-3 oil, from wild caught fish, and to eat no seafood at all. After three months, pathology tests came back clear, and I was able to ditch the medication. But mercury poisoning is also called *mad-hatters* disease. If he had not detected it, I would have been clinically insane years ago.

I hunted the vast inner landscapes, that are each of our personal mythos, for I don't know how long. I concluded—not incorrectly—that much of the martial arts so-called *government* was biased against me, without doubt, because I am woman. And this is, retrospectively and honestly, still the case. Even bodybuilding is still considered *a man's thing* by some.

I was angry, and I gave away much of my equipment or, in the case of uniforms and diplomas, ditched it all. I was tired, exhausted physically. Scared. Thinking about osteoporosis and seriously wondering if this was not the way of ageing after all.

I was both thin and not. I had this mass around my middle that I could not shift and a feeling, constantly, of bloating. I was still eating as I had done while training over the years, but had no idea what else to do. Except to starve myself.

Worth mentioning again: the bulge and discomfort, the bloating, was only around my middle and was not soft. I knew from my studies that this kind of fat deposit only comes from sugar... but I was only having one teaspoon in coffee or tea a couple of times day. Surely that could not be responsible? Turns out to be much more insidious.

Persistent research resulted in awareness of both the *Atkins* method of nutrition, and early research into Paleolithic eating. I am now paleo. Keto. I consume zero grains and zero sugar. That also means I must check the labeling of anything prepackaged when, or more likely if, I buy such.

4 GRAMS OF SUGAR AND A LUMP OF KILLER PLASTIC. HIDDEN POISONS

Beware the hidden sugars in canned tomatoes, beans, dozens of so-called healthy alternatives. I was daunted to know that a well-respected brand of bio-dynamic, organic tinned tomatoes contains 9 grams of sugar, with the addendum "No Added Sugar". That simply means that the preparation of preserving the ingredients has concentrated the fruit. This is not to suggest that the ancient tradition of harvesting and preserving is a no-no. That tradition is encouraged. It is wonderful if you have the wherewithal to do your own.

Sourcing what many producers call *uglies* is encouraged. These are fruit and vegetables that do not comply with a visual aesthetic. That's it. My local organic supplier sells large bags of *ugly* tomatoes, as well as turnips, squash, onions, you name it, for a song. I always buy them. Preserving is an art form and takes care and management, yes, but any library will stock appropriate titles, and many elder women are—thankfully—still alive and retaining the wisdom of this, from the grandmothers who u the healing arts. They will be able to advise you.

Most canned products, I must mention here, are lined with plastic. Plastic stiffened with BPA (Bisphenol-A) or an epoxy resin that utilizes BPA. What is it? An industrial chemical that has been used since the 1960s.

MORE ON BPA'S

Research has shown that this toxin can seep into food or beverages from containers that are made with BPA. pressure.

WHAT'S THE EVIDENCE ON BPA RISK?

While the research I have read is not conclusive nothing is worth the risk this chemical poses. Possible synthesis of BPA effects on the brain, and the behavior and prostate glands of fetuses, infants and children. Some research suggests a possible connection between BPA and increased toxicity.

While the jury is out, and if you are concerned—

- Look for products labeled as BPA-free. If a product is not labeled, keep in mind that some, but not all, plastics marked with recycle codes 3 or 7 may be made with BPA
- Reduce your use of canned foods since most are lined with BPA-containing resin
- Avoid heat. Don't microwave polycarbonate plastics or put them in your dishwasher. Plastic will break down over time and BPA will leach you're your food. Not only that but plastic breakdown is at pandemic proportions, both on land and at sea. An environmental catastrophe polluting everything and everyone
- Use glass, porcelain or stainless steel containers

What did I end up with? Learning this? Many of my recipes, and food-related topics are at *almostpaleocooking.wordpress.com*. I found nourishment. I realized how we are lied to by health authorities. That grains and sugars are inflammatory. That certain fats are absolutely necessary for optimum health. That the low-fat products I had been using in an attempt at healing my distressed gut, were, in fact, loaded with sugars.

I got to—and retain—a comfortable weight for my height of 160 cm. Fifty-four kilos. I train three days a week. I breathed away a healthy ten kilograms within three months of the change in both eating and cardio.

I now consume full fat everything: butter, lard, cream, cheese, as long as the cousins that produce these products have lived well, were grass fed, and were killed without fear. That have roamed. I check. I hunt down the food chain. Thankfully it is now common within certain sectors of the community for food providers to know this; to have source and researched their suppliers for themselves. It is now 'on trend' to graze on food from within a hundred kilometers of your home.

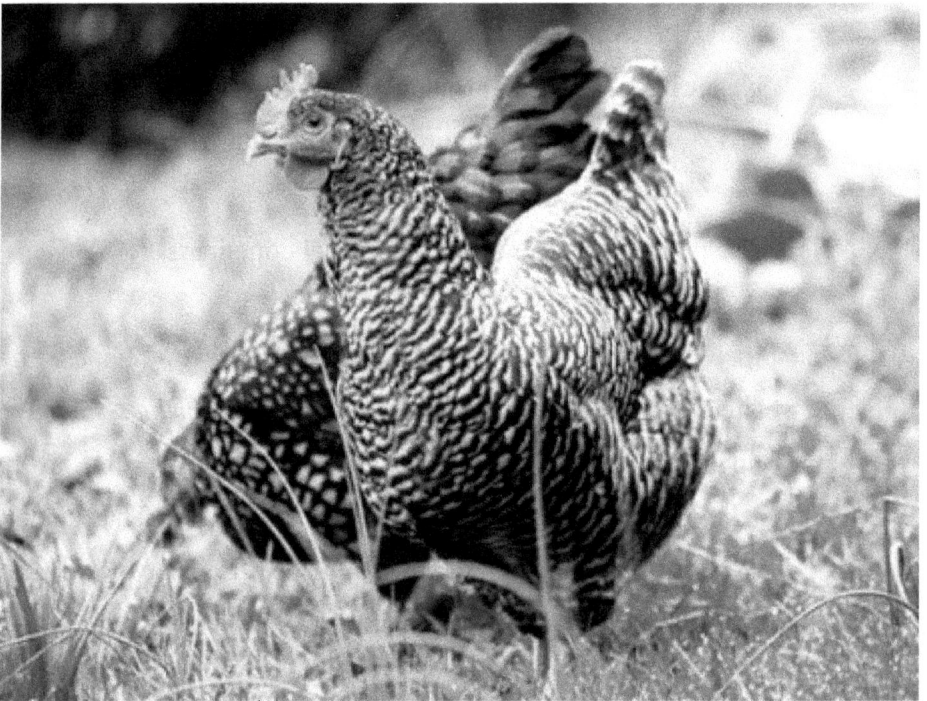

Do I pay more? A little. No point getting organic food that is grain-fed, even if the grain is organic. And although I consume quite a lot of fats I also eat large quantities of leaf and even edible weeds.

Protein? Every day. Small portions. Game meat, mostly.

VEGETABLES

And please buy organic wherever possible or grow them at home using good compost. And raw is best most of the time. All veggies that are cooked to where they lose their color and become floppy have lost everything. You will be eating dead food.

POTATOES: RARELY

Potatoes are high in starches and are complex sugars that supply long-term energy but—are they are high on the Glycemic Index[5]— and so I got rid of them. They are a fruit of the Andes and Chile, introduced to Europe by the Spanish invaders of those lands, and domesticated to the point whereby their demise, through fungal blight, resulted in the death of millions during the Irish Famine. But this is all also personal. Superphosphates, pesticides and aerial spraying of these crops almost killed my youngest son. Their use landed him in hospital as a two-year-old, because we lived behind a potato farm. He was allergic to the fine spray. What do these chemicals do to us? So, I'm rid of them. I occasionally roast pumpkin and parsnip and once or twice a week I will steam a yam or roast sweet potato of one variety or another.

All *colorful* vegetables are producers of what are called complex carbohydrates as well as minerals and vitamins that are deemed

---

[5] http://www.glycemicindex.com/

necessary for sustained health and vitality. They'll all give you fuel and you can eat them abundantly and you won't gain body fat.

Currently I'm residing in the Northern Rivers area of New South Wales, Australia. We get parasites from the water. From the rainwater, the creek, the water tank. Giardia, especially.

Organic brachia such as broccoli and cauliflower could harbor such things within their flowers so take preventative measures and just always think about this.

If you carefully collect and store your own water for drinking, you can reduce the risk of contamination by:

- Sealing your water storage so animals, birds and sunlight don't contaminate it
- Collecting water only from clean roofs, *not* from roofs that have been recently painted or painted with lead-based paints or coated with tar
- Installing fine-mesh screens on inlets and outlets to prevent mosquitoes breeding
- Cleaning your roof, gutters and water tanks regularly. If you can't do it for yourself, get a professional tank cleaner. Never enter a tank. Tanks are confined spaces and are very dangerous; the risks include loss of consciousness, asphyxiation and death
- Installing filters between the supply and storage
- Putting in a 'first flush' diversion device – the first rain after

a dry period contains most of the contaminants

- Ascertaining that surface run-off and leakage from sewage
- pipes and other drainage don't enter your water storage

OILS and FATS

Use only extra virgin cold extraction olive oil that has not been stored in light glass and is preferably of the first pressing. Macadamia oil, organic coconut oil, avocado oil or organic butter from grass-fed four-legged cousins. Ghee and even organic, quality lard.

All other oils and all *I-don't-believe-it's-not-butter* spreads are toxic. Please do not hurt yourselves with simple sugars and cheap, inexpensive fats. They are rancid and are stored as poisoned fat deposits.

All excess is EXCESS. Your energy input needs to be equal to your energy output to maintain a harmonious network between body and environment.

FRUIT

All fruit contains fructose. Fructose is a simple sugar. Fruit is good for gorillas. Seasonal fruit is best. In moderation. And don't ever juice it. How many oranges can you eat in one sitting?

WARNING: Fruit consumed just after a meal can ferment and you will experience extreme bloating. It is always best to eat fruit a few hours either side of any other kind of food, *especially* melon. Dried fruits are much higher in sugar content. Your choice, but know it. Fruit in cakes, breads, biscuits breakfast cereals or whatever, are going to load you with visceral white body fat.

PROTEIN:

MEAT, CHICKEN, FISH, EGGS

It bothers me that commercial farmers treat critter cousins with hormones and antibiotics, and it bothers me that they use chemicals and pesticides; that these cousins are forced to exist in cages or pens and know no freedom, that they are cruelly killed, called *chicken nuggets* without any awareness that they are the body-parts of once living baby birds, so I'm not going to eat that kind of flesh. Oh, I've got good reasons, and you should know about these things also, and I've already said enough. You won't need to go too far to your local bookstore, or to search the internet, to discover more.

Be that as it may, I eat flesh, and that includes rare, red meat. It contains creatine which translates within us into growth hormone – it's the only food that my research has found that will do so – and we are blessed, in Australia, to have wild kangaroos. They are hunted and shot, not farmed. Kangaroo and wallaby are lean and lacking the chemical abuse of commercially-imprisoned bovine, aquatic, feathered or *Babe*-styled little cousins in sow stalls. So cruel, and greedy.

I crave red meat when my blood-iron is low or when I have done extremely rigorous training. Women in so-called developed countries are debilitated, quite commonly, with iron deficiency. It causes extreme fatigue, listlessness and anxiety. These are also symptoms of estrogen-dominance as well as other dysfunctions. Get your bloods checked bi-annually, remembering that vitamin C is what transports iron through the body, so if taking a vitamin supplement of iron please do so in conjunction with 'C'.

I eat eggs daily. They are a much-maligned whole food. Again, from organic, pasture-fed, happy hens.

Seafood? Carefully, because of heavy metal poisoning, and over the past decade, mass pollution by plastic ingestion as well as over-fishing and the use of antibiotics in most fish farms. It's all getting a bit crazy. Calamari, prawns, NZ mussels, crab. Lightly cooked, 3 minutes in water with lemon used as a seasoning. Throw in some ginger, maybe chili, carrot, bean sprouts. Eat on a cold green salad; serve it with steamed greens. Just remember Fukushima nuclear reactor, damaged in the earthquake of '11, is still leaching radiation into the circulation system of Mother Earth's oceanic highways, second by second. It's like poker.

GRAINS

I do not eat grains. I DO NOT EAT GRAINS.

ESSENTIAL FATS

I repeat, we need certain kinds and qualities of oils and fats to ensure good health. There are fatty acids derived from fish, the pressings from avocados, sesame seeds (tahini or sesame oil, not the seeds themselves), pure virgin first crop cold-extracted olive, evening primrose oil.

Essential fats, in seeds and nuts, only remain wholesome for a short shelf-life. When they have been exposed to light and oxygen for any length of time they become stale (sometimes moldy) and rancid. And that rancidity is toxic. Carcinogenic Ascertain that all are kept in airtight containers away from light, and always buy oils in dark bottles. Preferably gather nuts in the shell and crack them open when you are ready to eat them.

This is not a detailed analysis of foods, however, but what you will understand, by now, is that you are to eat for happiness and health. And for the future of wisdom. Hey, people you know, or meet in the future, are going to need to know what you do now. This is healing work passed along. So, the simpler the variety of flora that you can consume the better, especially if it's palatable raw or *just* cooked and the greener, fresher-picked the better, as chlorophyll and the attending nutriments of leafy greens and sprouts are roughage necessity. Like cats and dogs eating.

In June of 2018 alfalfa sprouts from one South Australian company poisoned many people with salmonella. It had happened previously, in 2012. Enough to make me think twice about buying commercial brands.

Magic requires intense consciousness. Choosing and preparing food is a decisive act of sorcery. Art and magic. You enter communion with what is consumed. You become *one*. Eating is a ceremony of earthy profundity.

Lettuce (all varieties), cucumber, parsley, basil, dill, rocquette, coriander, avocados, oriental greens, spinach, all sprouted vegetables, watercress, shallots, fennel, spinach, Warangal greens, purslane, bush tucker foods (in Australia).

And eat them all.
And eat them raw.

Tomatoes, chili, beetroot, carrots, red capsicum, red onion, garlic. You can eat all this raw or you can, I suppose, if you must, cook it. You'll want legumes in moderation, if at all. You might want a variety of sea vegetables, and organic tomato paste/puree. Just please be aware that several in this list are nightshades and, if you have a gut reaction, discard them as part of your regime.

Bio-dynamic yogurt (I prefer goat or sheep), full cream cottage or cream cheese, full cream organic pasture-fed cow, goat or sheep milk. Organic sour cream, Butter. Lard from healthy free range animal people.

Peas and snow-peas, mushrooms, broccoli, cauliflower, cabbage, asparagus, radish, squash, turnip, pumpkin. Spinach and kale, mizuna and bok choy, and any/all dark leafy greens. Any time. You can eat most of them raw or you can steam, blanch, bake, fry, make soup, casserole, anything. And eggs. Did I mention eggs?

Anything eaten should be enjoyable. If it's boring, it's boring. If it's tasteless, it's tasteless. If it's colorless, it's colorless. What you eat, and how you have prepared food reflects the creative, intelligent, beautiful, careful, passionate, obstinate, focused, respectful, detailed, determined and honest you. Magic.

Eating is so *necessary*. It is as exciting as good comedy, as learning witchery with friends, as a swim in hot weather, as a cozy fire when it's cold and dreary, as surprising as an unexpected gift for no other reason than that someone really likes you. As when a rain dance invokes brother thunder.

Remember that we have this reptilian reward-center in our brains, and we must be mindful of self-indulgence. The more you reward yourself the quicker the slide into obesity or any other addiction. Either that or you have parasites living, breeding and dying in your gut. Forgot to mention this. A check up for that will not be a waste of money.

SUPPLEMENTS

Where supplements are concerned in any discussion of good health it is to be noted that you are to go, first last and always for live food and to the supplementation of vitamins and minerals as just that.

Research different articles concerning the necessity or lack thereof relative to supplementation. It can get confusing. A bio-chemist, years ago, suggested that her thesis had concluded that when we take lots of supplements our bodies become reliant on them and will not produce them naturally from what we eat. The depletion of soils[6], however, the use of pesticides and fertilizer for decades, often over a lifetime, have done what? Is our food adequate when training or working very hard? Lifting and carrying? Unable to afford organic? I don't think that's true anymore. It's twenty years since that idea was discussed. What is agriculture now? Many questions need to be asked of the food industries today. Too many for this work. I'll have the supplements. When I train I consume B.C.A.A.'s (Branch Chain Amino Acids) and *I do* heal faster than I would otherwise, and I do a better workout. Check on, and compare, the brands.

Be careful of hype and hidden sugars/chemicals. Currently I use ATP Science *NOWAY* Protein because it is such a well-researched product.

I take anti-oxidants. COQ10 in the form of Ubiquinol Forte. How can I tell that their use is not a placebo? Well, you never know, really, but I don't get sick, and my vitality is high most of the time.

---

[6] See *World Ending Fire*, the Essential Wend all Berry, 2019

___

Stress doesn't get to me as much anymore unless I'm around toxic people for too long or scroll Facebook for more than a minute. Calcium, zinc and magnesium are all necessary. You could, I suppose, take a supplement but you'll get these minerals from eating abundant alfalfa and sprouted seeds. Potassium from bananas.

I'm a productive, driven human and I can be horrible when I'm hungry. To be healthy I learned that I didn't have get to the stage of being on empty to be depleted, as lack of food has nothing to do our stomachs but, rather, the mitochondria (nuclear-powered generators), in each cell.

Since choosing to go full paleo, almost carnivore, I do not feel hungry. I will, on some days, have two eggs in the morning, kale and broccoli poached in butter and either high quality free-range bacon or left-overs. Other days I have ground nuts, seed, walnuts and raw yogurt. Sparingly as I'm aware of oddities like diverticulitis, a disorder many people suffer from as a result of consumption of too many nuts, seeds and whole grains. They can cause pockets in the average fifteen feet of hairpin-bend intestine and that can then cause popping, like herniation, even infection. The few people I have learned from, who suffer with this, live terrified lives. On my website click the drop-down menu for Body/Mind/Spirit. That will take you to my blog where I have recorded many easily prepared, delicious, tried-and-true recipes and anecdotal articles.

Occasionally I'll make certain that I have cassoulet'd enough for the following morning or I would have cooked a cauliflower and a fennel bulb together, sautéed in butter sourced from grass-fed cows, blended them, added Dijon mustard, cayenne pepper, a hinted dash of nutmeg and good quality grated cheese. I would have had that for dinner with a dark leafy green salad and a slab of wallaby the night before. In the morning it is always tastier, and I will put it in a pan with an egg and heat it till the albumin is white. I'll squeeze on lemon juice and serve it with avocado slices over a bed of fresh rocquette from my garden.

LOW BLOOD SUGAR

When glycogen is low the sensation is *Body-death, body-death! Immanent body-death!* (even though you can't understand the language the signs are obvious). You have exhausted your previous intake of nutrition and will need to eat again, even if the meal you take is small. I recommend making up a few meatball treats the night before as these will get you through the doldrums.

Depression, anxiety and aggression are often caused by hunger or ineffective nutrition. SO, FUEL UP WELL.

PYRROLE DISORDER?

Then there are times when you won't be able to get 'up' no matter how happy you are, no matter what you eat, no matter how well you are resting. That's often the result of relationship dysfunction or other anxieties so prevalent in the current world of pollution (of so many different kinds, even psychological). Life sometimes takes it out of you. Suggestion? Be clear and change what needs changing. And get a check-up. You could be B or D deficient. Or be experiencing pyroluria. Pyroluria is considered genetic but so are lots of things, like hypertension, when it's actually generations of stress that passes to you via an inherited trauma—intergenerational—whatever. The glitch can also strike you through stress and environmental pollutants. I live with it. The symptoms of pyrrole disorder are

- White spots on fingernails
- Hypoglycemia/sugar intolerance (common and is sometimes referred to as Jekyll and Hyde personality)
- Food and environmental allergies
- Joint pain
- Fatigue (often unexplained)
- Irritable bowel, constipation, gut pain and distention
- Dizziness
- Dizziness
- Insomnia
- Insomnia
- Poor memory and concentration
- A lack of stress control
- Poor emotional regulation - episodic anger, or depression, may seem manic at times
- ADHD

Who among you is reading this and *thinking, this is me*. There is relief. I use Pyrrole Protect by the company *BioCeuticals*. Takes a couple of days to notice but there IS noticeable relief.

WOMEN AND HORMONES

Firstly, if you go to a sports physician and explain that you're doing resistance training (or whatever endurance training you're doing) and that you're experiencing some continuous fatigue you can get broad-range blood tests to find out whether you are deficient in one of many things (you also get the benefits of cholesterol testing and discovering whether your white blood count is appropriate). Get tested once or twice a year to be on the safe side.

Secondly: if you are a cis woman, thirty-five years or over, you are in perimenopause. If you are still fatigued, it's quite likely that you are progesterone deficient. Progesterone (outside the body) is a naturally derived substance produced from wild yam.

Through a process of fermentation, the little mother synergizes with a female human-animal body. The liver breaks down any ingested form of progesterone-producing foods, and so the only way you'll benefit (and benefit you will) is to topically apply the cream *Progest*, or whatever brand you buy, where it is taken up by the small vascular system. Profound life-changing effects are reported in a wide variety of its users, including me. It is even reported, in the relevant documentation, to reverse osteoporosis.

Over 40? Hard-core mood swings begin what idiots call mid-life crisis. It's not. It's hormonal *koyaanisqatsi*. After 50/55, menopause will have you believing that the church was right. There is a male god. And he hates women. There are now many ways of rethinking what can be extremely traumatic so hunt for yourselves. For me, yes, these were the weird years because so little science takes women into account unless we can be sold on some drug or another. We will, however, be told (by now) that we are, as mentioned earlier, *unfuckable*. These are the years to use this to our own advantage. To hear ourselves. To get back to who we were before we lost our *shine*.

Over the past several decades only, xenoestrogens[7], a synthetic that mimics phytoestrogens have markedly reduced the effectiveness of naturally-occurring progesterone. This has resulted in a deficiency that can quite radically decrease the quality of life of most women in the so-called developed world, and as toxins are stored in body fat there is now one more urgent reason for change.

What is happening instead?

An obesity epidemic of epic scale, most of which is caused by the intake of sugars, processed foods and an increasing lack of exercise, is currently a commodification warzone. Made more existential by too much sitting. Synthesized estrogens—these insidious chemical

---

[7]https://womeninbalance.org/2012/10/26/xenoestrogens-what-are-they-how-to-avoid-them/

compounds—are fed to factory animals as well as leaching into our environment from a currently incalculable number of cosmetics, food additives, pesticides, herbicides and common household products. In men xenoestrogens are known to decrease, or even destroy, fertility. Ditto in women, with the tragedy of increased cancers. Extensive research is up to you, but it is very worth taking the time to understand some of the data to be able to make lifestyle choices.

GROWTH HORMONE IN FOOD

A salmon that grows to market size twice as fast as normal. Dairy cows that produce 15% more milk. Beef cows that grow 20% faster. What do these hyper-productive animals have in common? Thanks to injections and implants (in the case of cows) or genetic engineering (in the case of salmon), they contain artificially high levels of sex or growth hormones. Are these hormones dangerous to the humans who eat the food or drink the milk? [8]

All I can suggest is that you avoid it all. That we join the movements and activism against the artificial interference of multinationals and biased food and drug administrations, to demand accountability. We want to consider the harm. Unfortunately, we must remain suspicious and vigilant. As ever. We have been done in before by

---

[8] https://www.health.com/health/article/0,,20458816,00.html

governments and authorities. Other than Hypatia and Veronica Franco many—mostly—women across Europe and into America, were tortured and/or killed. For what? Supposedly for witchcraft.

Did you know that before the Scottish bloke, James the First, had his biblical texts translated into English there was an obscure word, mekhashepha, that could have meant one of dozens of titles? Poisoner is, today, thought the most common (an effective means of doing away with a king, which is why they all had tasters). Jimmy, however, had been brought up to hate independent women. Herbalists, midwives, those who wouldn't allow his rape, so when he had the opportunity to mistranslate the word *mekhashepha* to *witch*, he jumped at the chance. This was the era of far right christianity and the violent persecution of anyone in denial and defiance of an establishment with a fetish for everything devilish and demonic.

Oh wait… that's over? No one told us, did they?

In 1597, James felt sufficiently knowledgeable about witchcraft that he wrote *"Daemononlogie"*. This was an eighty-page book that expounded his views on the topic and it was meant to add to the intellectual debate that was going on within Europe about witchcraft. The book has three sections on magic, sorcery and witchcraft and one on spirits and ghosts. Having produced this book, James decided to end the standing commission that had been established to hunt out witches. However, the persecution did not end. By the time he left for England in 1603, witches were still being arrested and of those arrested, half were executed. Between 1603 and 1625, there were about twenty witchcraft trials a year in Scotland – nearly 450 in total.

Half of the accused were found guilty and executed.

The above is an abridged version of accounts. No one mentions oleander, toadstools and voluptuous quantities of henbane in the histories. Let alone poverty, and the weather and a hemorrhage after the botched abortion on the kitchen table.

A recent study by Maria Dominguez-Bellow at *New York University School of Medicine*[9] theorizes that C-section babies are more likely to become fat. This study suggests that a caesarean section prevents newborns from the coating of bacteria they would otherwise receive from a vaginal birth, and that would typically establish themselves in a baby's gut, thereby improving future health. The conclusion is that, while a connection between obesity and the types of bacteria living in someone's gut is well established, the way in which it comes about is still open to debate.

Dominguez-Bellow's is attempting to discover whether it is the procedure itself that keeps the baby and bacteria apart or the large amounts of antibiotics typically administered with surgery. The study aims to determine whether caesarean sections are to blame for promoting bacteria-mediated obesity. According to several sources up to 20% of American babies are delivered by caesarean section, but a staggering 32% in Australia, and up to 42% in private hospitals[10]. In some instances, this technique will save a life, sure, but in most cases? Expediency. The dangers are becoming more apparent over the years.

BODYBUILDING, WITCHCRAFT, HEALING

What has any of this got to do with bodybuilding, witchcraft and healing? Everything if you have no choice in the matter of your own health, that of your family, friends and earthly community. And especially if you title yourself a healer and are working with the lives of others. Ask your mother how you arrived. Think of Lorenzo's Oil[11]. Do we really want to rely on answers to our overall health and well-being to a bunch of people who never learned about nutrition and exercise in their many years of study? Who would rather charge money for surgery than have a golf game interrupted? Better to trust midwives. They have more knowledge of pregnancy, birth and post-natal care in their little fingers than most doctors have from every textbook they'll ever read? They used to burn us for thinking they knew better.

Or lock us up in Bedlam. Or prescribe us lots of pharmaceutical drugs to shut us up. Or down. Or in. Or off. Or out.

---

[9] (http://advances.sciencemag.org/content/3/10/eaao1874.full)
[10] (https://www.bellybelly.com.au/birth/why-australias-c-section-rate-is-so-high/)
[11] https://en.wikipedia.org/wiki/Lorenzo%27s_Oil

I AM

STRONG
POWERFUL
FEARLESS
HAPPY
HOPEFUL
AMAZING
LOVING
THANKFUL
BLESSED

Dear Diary,

What screws with my desire to listen is...

Have I explained that amino acids are PROTEIN? Protein heals us.
We are made up, bodily, of proteins, water, sugars and minerals.
What we don't need (false food) are simple sugars;
monocarbohydrates.

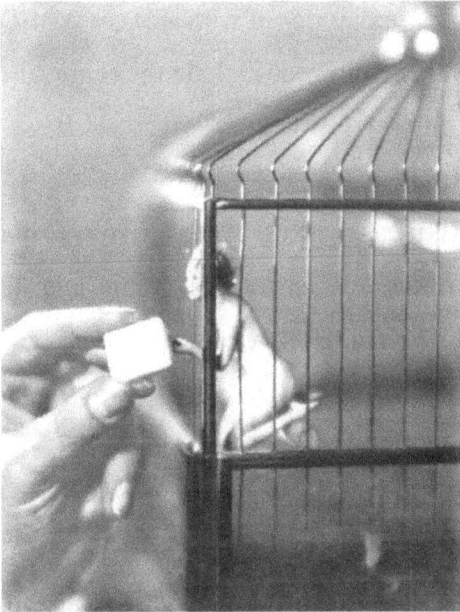

They are not food and are toxic to our organ function. Mainly the
pancreas and the weird effect that they produce relative to the
resultant insulin response. You are fooled into thinking you are
being fed. Sugars and carbohydrates are fat-making. Only in the
instance of insulin production and the benefits of this (an entire other
study, see *Insulin and the Insulin Spike,* p 49). Within a short period
of time of consumption, you'll flat line, and will crave more of the

same, as it gets used up so quickly without any fulfillment other than being pleasant to your taste buds.

I wonder whether this addiction is to the intoxicant or the sugar. Or both. Some people have reported violent behavior at the hands of out-of-control alcoholics.

Often people who are hyperactive, are diagnosed with ADD or ADHD and whose diet, if the problem was recognized, include the removal of all sugars and additives[12]The same with wheat.

If you cannot get off other grains, please get off wheat (*Grain Brain* by David Perlmutter, Kristin Loberg). It is not only toxic and an opiate, but also highly addictive and an aggressive inflammatory.

> *"Researchers have known for some time now that the cornerstone of all degenerative conditions, including brain disorders, is inflammation. ...."*
> ~~David Perlmutter, *Grain Brain: The Surprising Truth about Wheat, Carbs, and Sugar—Your Brain's Silent Killers*

Don't over-eat BUT eat to satisfaction. Small meals, eaten regularly speed the metabolism in a healthy body.

...

---

[12] https://www.additudemag.com/adhd-diet-nutrition-sugar/

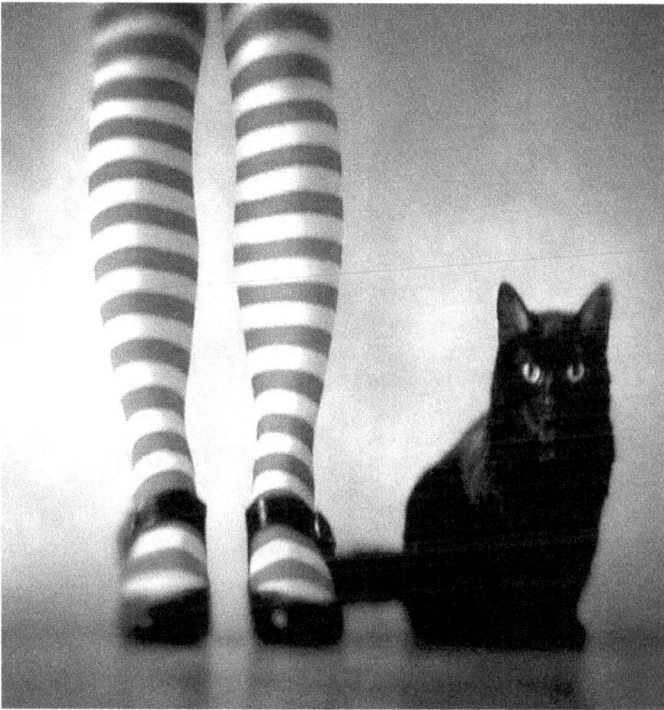

Dear Diary,

I speak to spirits and call them *god*. What I understand that to be is...

Enormous pyres, built over days, by big, strong blokes. Fires of an epic proportion burn at the very sliver of a snow-crunchy dawned, Midwinter Solstice, revered by a crowd that will feast the day away, be drunk on so many hopes, such friendship, such knowledge of an inherited alignment with earth. Kids building cubbies and making crow wing shapes in the snow.

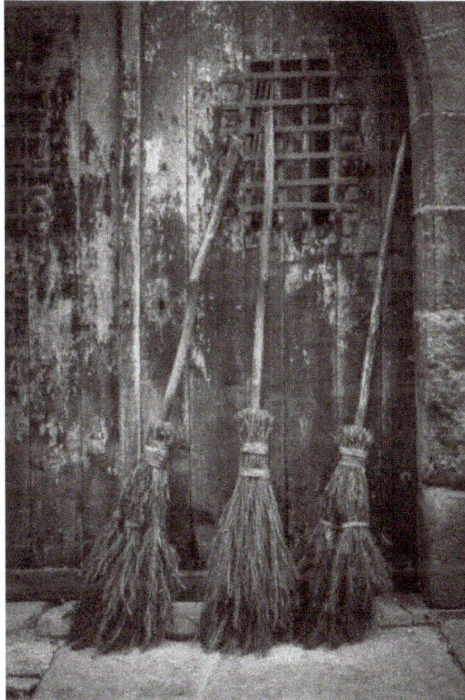

For the courageous, the mystics and the crazy, there's the crop of gold-top mushrooms dancing in a circle around the base of a whopping great pine, planted by some European interloper, generations-long dead, nostalgic to not have to look at one more eucalypt tree, so alien to the limbic brain entrenched in the landscapes of ancestry: used to skies less blue, moreso in winter.

Afternoons the fires continue in slow combustion stoves and open hearths and the young piper is the Pied Piper, stealing all the rugged up children. He is over on that grassy knoll, in the thickest fog since custard, playing a bagpipe air that will summon tears from farmers living miles away. This will become legend in the pubs of Castlemaine within days. The cycles of earth bring the smells of long ago, and with them the dead who live, yet, beneath stars.

...

RELATIONSHIPS AND THEIR PITFALLS

Not all food is necessarily either edible or nourishing, but quite often we do not realize it until it's in our mouths or causing tragedy to our guts. Non-edible, non-nourishing, also, is the kind we interact with, touch or are touched by: psychic, empathic, affecting, infecting, infesting our lives, emotionally non-essential, or unjust. Relationships, in other words.

Relationships can feed or poison us. I have spoken and written on this subject many times but because the afflicted keep coming to me, clients and friends, witches, wildlings, widely-differing gender people, lawyers and sex workers, women or men both old and young, their early-adult offspring, people from a multitude of ethnic and cultural complexities. Those who have trained as healers. Because the problem of dysfunction never seems to go away it, also, must be understood. And almost from an intergenerational perspective. People have been taught lies.

The follow-your-dream trope is rubbish—a modern-day trope—as very often dreams seem to make no sense at all, or can as easily be nightmares. Do those sprouting this actually mean aspirations. Happiness? About what to expect and what is expected within all relationships, from those with a parent or employer, from your lover to a teacher, across the entire socio-economic spectrum of the so-called industrialized world. The taint stemming from a privileged, colonial Anglo-European, androcentric and Abrahamic religious ideology.

LOVE OR CHEMISTRY?

FOREVER

To what am I referring? Love, as an interactive, at least. Do I think there is such a thing as love? I don't know. It is an elusive, and enigmatic concept. Or even a construct.

Oh, horror, you poor thing, you might think. But hear me out. An article I wrote a while back is added here for your consideration, before I provide you a breakdown of why I think there is no such thing. And that yearning for something that is a construct of the movie and music industry, the lingerie industry and others who will benefit financially from the theory. Trusting love is forever, when everything changes naturally, is fool's gold. Believing in love, demanding it or living without it are concepts that will drive you to despair. Sooner or later.

I do not know what love is. I experience a vast forest of sensations and responses, of which I am, and you are, and we are. Where there's no road, so no road-kill, no in and no out. But is any of this love? Or is that just what we say when we have nothing to explain? Oh, and those who think to try to tell me? To think to help this old witch to know what I ought, by now, to know? Why, I'm the nightmare, then, of you being lost in said forest, and not knowing what love is, after all. Of looking for the road that has cut you into this side or that. And there's the answer. If you try, you're already lost. (Ly de Angeles, 2016)

I want to be honest with you. If I lie to you about this how can you trust anything I write? So, here we go.

Love = interactive, empathic collaboration, coupled with affection, and in mating instances, with desire, or lust. Without the latter two we have any type of relationship from a job to riding a horse. That's the beginning, like the blush of the first peach to ripen on the tree. A parent's first cuddle with their newborn child, a lover's first kiss, a child's first friend, opening the box in which is a bundle of fur called a puppy. The affection aspect can change. To apathy, to disdain. Contempt, often just below the surface of acquiescence through learned behavior, not new data. How is that love? It is not.

A new series of emotive responses replace affection. They can be obedience, triggered by a reward/denial continuum, obligation, a habit-induced behavioral modality very often present, in parents (usually induced by religious and cultural stereotypes) and the wife/husband syndrome of ownership. Empathy dies or is disrupted when an essential predisposition or indoctrination to the constructed ideology of superiority and/or authority is recognized as just that—a construct.

This is the bases of personal and cultural revolution. Like the scales of the mythic dragon lifting from our eyes. The true nature of these anomalies may very well have been suppressed, initially, by the release on both parties, of the feel-good, desire-nurture hormone oxytocin—the hormone that triggers an amorous sensation of bonding. The innate tendency of an individual/animal to, at certain life stages, attempt to wrest an alpha position in a pack, herd, flock, family or relationship is misunderstood. Misinterpreted.

To try to retain a misplaced dominance, the human animal will become judgmental, the all-knowing advice-giver, will presume the role of the greater, or more personally significant, person. Get their kicks from conspiracy theories in order to fill the sadness of loss.

ISOLATION

The *opposite* of that initial interactive, empathic collaboration, coupled with affection (generalized by the word *love*), is isolation. Often accompanied by shame. To remain in a toxic relationship is to become ill. Your gut will inform you. You will become either fat or wasted. You will wither at the core of you.

Physical healing restores well-being. It is a cure for depression and anxiety, both of which, when not chemically-induced, are the response of the illusion of love being instilled, then debased. Understand that another kind of food/nourishment is oxytocin.

MACRO/MICRO SYMBIOTIC HEALTH

How did our relatives know the difference between an edible fungus, a deadly one and the kind that alters our perception of reality and teaches us the nature of the mysticism that both surrounds us and of which we are an integral part? How did our relatives discover what heals and what kills? To ingest this, smoke that? Was it trial and error? I somehow do not think so.

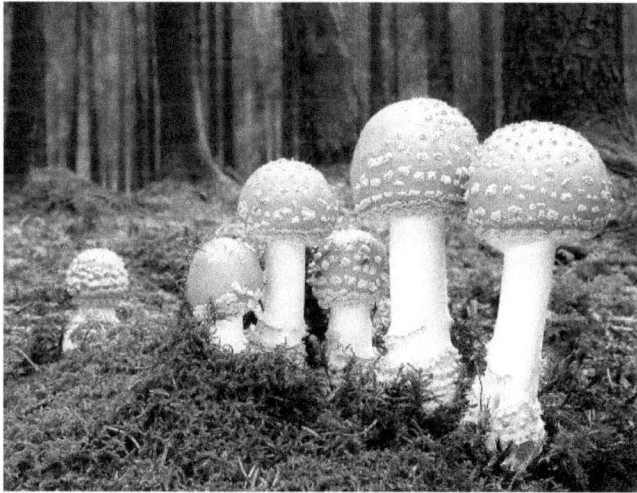

Consider, that prior to the human animal having had its forever-skills most universally obfuscated through the terror of both religious brainwashing and mass killing, we lived a symbiotic relationship with other life-forms and that we did not objectify as we do now. We did not perceive the earth as us and/or *it*.

Sometimes at odds with *it*.

Two things to wonder about:

Kambo is the venomous secretion of PHYLLOMEDUSA BICOLOR (the giant leaf or monkey frog), a bright green tree frog native to the Amazon basin. It can be found in the rainforest regions of northern Brazil, eastern Peru, southeastern Colombia, and parts of Venezuela, Bolivia, and the Guianas. In many regions outside Brazil, both the frog and its secretion are known as SAPO, or toad.

Kambo has a range of traditional and potential therapeutic applications, both medical and psycho-spiritual. Commonly described as an 'ordeal medicine', the secretion is known for its powerful emetic or purgative effects. Despite its initial unpleasantness, kambo is widely sought out to revitalize body and mind.

Hallucinogenic species of the Psilocybe genus have a history of use among the native peoples of Mesoamerica for religious communion, divination, and healing, from pre-Columbian times to the present day.

They are found in Australia in cow pastures, and, in the southern states, in pine forests at the time of the first frosts, probably shipped to the southern continent at the time of European settlement.

Cultures prize certain animals and plants as aphrodisiacs, as life-extenders, as fertility-inducing and as a natural abortive. My curiosity has never been sated. Who decided these things? How, as with the giant Peruvian tree frog producing kambo, did someone know to spread the frog's legs between four sticks to stress into activation the secretion of the potentially deadly toxin? To burn the skin before application? That it would enhance eyesight in the jungle? How did the medicine people learn this? Unless through a form of mutual and symbiotic relationship?

How did the fungus ergot, mold on the rye in damp and swampy soils, become associated with witchcraft? Why was it responsible for the murder of so many when, in the twentieth century, its properties became the core of psychological experiments, and is known as LSD?

I theorize that the human animal is in symbiosis with internal and external biology always and, whether bacteria, microwaves or THC we can be aware of this. Only then can we choose to relate to other species in a respectful and harmonious manner. Only then can the process of health and well-being be mutually meaningful, both microcosmically and in the wider senses, macrocosmically.

I definitely recommend the studies of Paul Stamets and Wade Davis in relation to matters of forest and field medicine. Doctor Stamets speaks with Joe Rogan on YouTube at #1035. It's a fascinating hour.

...

Dear Diary,

I have never felt as alive as when ...

REPEAT AFTER ME—

SOMETIMES I PRETEND TO BE NORMAL.

but it gets boring.

SO I GO BACK TO Being me.

There are no answers, only questions.

Keeps you free, knowing that.

...

There are two
rules in life:
1. Never give out
all the information

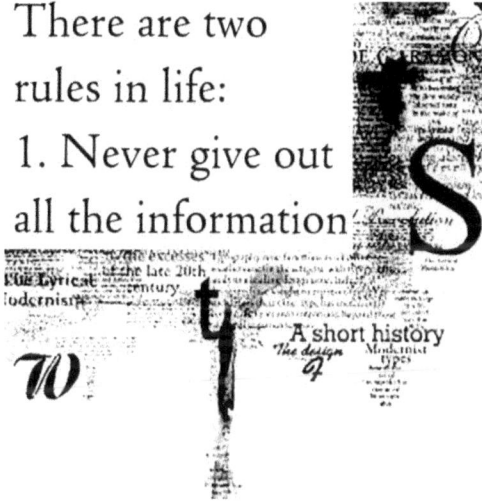

- You need not do all these exercises in one session
- Anything else you will discover with continual training and observation. Anything you need to know; please ask someone you are SURE knows
- Reject others' concepts of limit. Get to know, for yourself, what you can achieve. Not age, not sex, not current body-state is a problem. There are always solutions to what gives you grief
- OLD CODGER = Coffin Dodger

...

PREY

TASTES LIKE DEPRESSION, LOOKS LIKE SELF DOUBT, FEELS LIKE BETRAYAL

Scary days are the ones when that beast lies in stealth between your groin and my gut. It's the threat of insignificance or failure with an almost, not quite, silent breath of loneliness.

You purposely ignore it because if you look it in the eye you know it'll go you; go for the throat. You ignore it until something in the day distracts you or you can outdistance it.

It seems then, that it retreats back into its lair until it can sneak up on you again. It's like being haunted. Like you're still 15; like you're the prey of your own ghost.

We all know it. We share a commonality. We are it. But, I reserve the right to go off at a tangent…

FERAL

…what defines *wild* from *tame*? Cannot the four-legged companion have chosen life with you?

This presumption of *bestiality* being crude or vile really requires a second thought. So does the word *brutal*. As does the word *savage*, as does the word *feral*.

People are all of the above. When we are not intentionally violent or cruel.

...

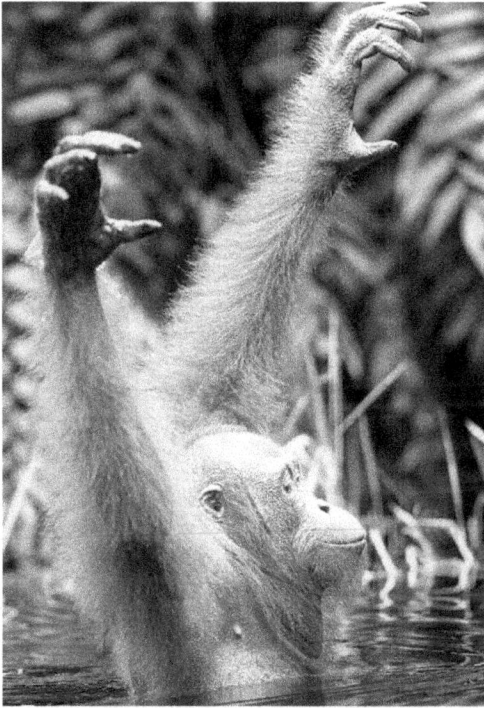

Image: theanimal-zone.blogspot.com

ORANGUTANS AND SPORT WINNERS

In the so-described developed countries a crisis, unrelated to food or lack of exercise, is having a huge impact on future health. That is the mobile phone and the computer screen/keyboard

HARMING THE FUTURE ONE SLOUCH AT A TIME

I often live in Melbourne, Australia, and travel by public transport, often, rather than by car. Everyone, in trams and trains and buses, on the street, walking and sitting and eating, is bent over their mobile devices reading, shopping or playing something. Two things are occurring:

1. The language of this posture is despair.

2. An adult human head weighs between 10 and 12 pounds. As it tilts or angles forward, the cervical spine's (neck) muscles, tendons, and ligaments that support the head during movement and when static are engaged; such as holding the head in a forward tilted position. Even the neck's intervertebral discs are involved and help absorb and distribute the forces exerted on the neck. The use of these devices affects your posture, contributing to neck, upper back, shoulder, and arm pain. Furthermore, poor posture while sitting, standing, walking, or in a static position can lead to more than upper body disease and stiffness—poor posture affects other aspects of the us, right down the spine, including the nervous system, affecting the sciatic, knees and, ultimately all of us

I see parents with toddlers in prams, or playing in the park, anywhere really, and the adults are on their phones. No social interaction with the young advises that body-to-body, eye-to-eye contact is abnormal. Do you see the future? This redisposition to a lack of body and verbal communication is causing depression. Isolation. All those symptoms I mentioned in the chapter on a lack of love. Without the capacity to read a body danger is exponential and intimacy threatened.

LIFTING THE STERNUM, WHAT COULD BE EASIER?

Necessary to bodybuilding, but also to all aspects of health, is postural integrity. Remembering, regularly, to merely lift your sternum, consciously, aligns the entire spine. That and a straight head, as though an invisible thread is pulling the center of the skull skyward.

AMY CUDDY: FAKE IT TILL YOU MAKE IT

Amy Cuddy is an American social psychologist, author and speaker. She became well known for her 2012 TED talk, presenting research on body language.

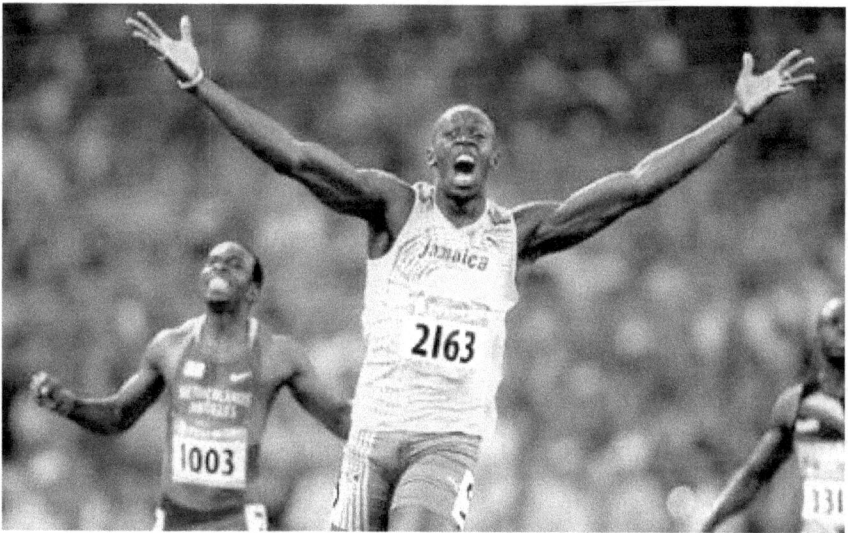

Image: Usain Bolt 2012 Olympic 200 meter winner

Cuddy has done work on stereotyping and discrimination, emotions, nonverbal behavior, and the effects of social stimuli on hormone levels.

When we scrutinize ourselves, we think about how other people are judging us. We're not wrong to do so.

"We make sweeping judgments and inferences from body language," and those judgments can predict enormously important life outcomes. What do humans do? The same thing. They stretch out.

When you walk or stand tall, your inner organs are comfortable, there is no pressure on your lower back, your gall bladder is draining well, your intestines are processing information unimpeded, there is no strain on your neck. *The knee-bone's connected to the thighbone.*

This opening of the *dantian*—the lifting of the sternum—is a primal body language that speaks volumes. Any primate, or species-cousin for that matter, that has no fear, need not cover the belly or the throat. We are strong enough and sufficiently trained/prepared to defend ourselves or others.

Yes, it can be seen as a challenge. But only when we overextend the information: jut the chin. Opening the arms sideways (while jutting the chin) in a seeming-welcome gesture, summoning an opponent. Dropping the chin is inviting an embrace.

Hands on hips, toes pointing towards each other instead of straight ahead? Head tilted to one side? Bent shoulders as though walking into a gale? One or two fists raised in the air? Big stories. No need for words.

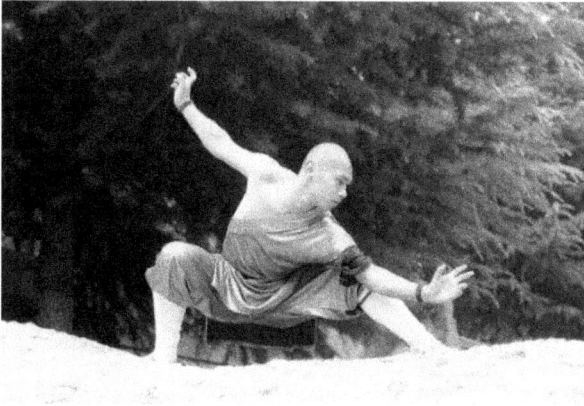

Nancy Brown/Photolibrary/Getty Images

I stood at a music venue, around the age of 60, in a usual crowd, spread-legged, arms crossed over my chest, and a woman came up to me asking if I was security. What does that tell you? A police officer will come too close to your face if interrogating you. A lover will do the same if readying to kiss you. It's an intimate, claiming gesture. Seated at a dinner with half a dozen people and someone sits just that tiny bit too close. You are threatened and intimidated.

UNTO THE 7TH GENERATION

Your entire life, which in the case of this book includes healing through bodybuilding—strength and agility, is super important. Reclaim your entire life.

Do you even realized you have lived untaught? The *7th Generation* philosophy is commonly credited to the Iroquois Confederacy but practiced by many Native nations. This philosophy mandates that decision-makers consider the effects of their actions and agreements for descendants seven generations into the future.

There is a clear understanding that everything we do has consequences for something and someone else, reminding us that we are intimate threads in the web of all life.

Body/earth relationship is a vast network of intra-universal communications. What are we adding to the conversation?

...

SCARLET WOMAN?

ON SEXUAL FULFILLMENT AND HYPOCRISY

scarlet woman

Meaning—

noun

a sexually promiscuous woman, especially a prostitute or a woman who commits adultery.

a symbol of pagan Rome or, derogatorily, of the church of Rome[13].

OLD WOMEN IN RED DRESSES

(Cloch na Rón—Roundstone—County Connemara, Ireland 2006)

In my dream four old women walk around a large square pit lurid with chemical turquoise water, far below in its depths. The women go for tea at an outdoor table with four chairs and an umbrella flapping at its center. The oldest woman, at the rear of the group, is dressed all in red and carries a red brolly. She's forgotten something. She walks back the way she has come but is dangerously close to the edge of the pit.

"No!" I scream. "Look out!"

Being a dream, of course, she doesn't hear me. I watch, impotent and in horror, as the edge crumbles away. In slo-mo she crashes into the

---

[13] https://www.dictionary.com/browse/scarlet-woman

alien-colored pit and drowns. Flip, and it's years later and legend circulates amongst locals that a scarlet demon dwells in that pit and I see a lovely young guy amble down the well-worn track to the water at its base. He carries a posy of flowers to appease the demon (or perhaps make a wish).

In less time than it takes to blink, the scarlet demon explodes from the water, grabs him and drags him under. Then I wake up and tell my traveling companion. As we discuss it we realize there's actually no old women on the street—there's only one street—in Roundstone.

So we walk up the stairs of the art gallery where I'll be launching the pre-release of *THE QUICKENING*, to Sheena Keene, my host, who is drinking coffee, sitting in her office chair.

"Where are all the old women?" I ask.

"Oh, they don't come out. They're widows."

I'm a bit disturbed by this as you can imagine. "Why are they all widows?

"Fishermen. The sea takes 'em." She sips her coffee like this is a normal conversation. I tell her about the dream.

Doesn't matter that no one's got an interpretation because later in the day we're in a grocery shop and a woman, maybe 85 or 90 years old and all in black—widow's weeds, I suppose—tiny and bent, comes into the shop on the arm of a middle aged man. And she looks at me. And ponders. Her scrutiny lasts maybe thirty seconds. It's an uncomfortable moment but she breaks the stalemate. She comes right up to me and stares me in the eye.

"I'm lookin' at de look," she says. I smile. "Do you mind dat I'm lookin' at de look?" She's brazen. I appreciate that.

"Nah, I don't mind," I say.

She walks around me. Takes her time. Touches my arm; my tattooed hand. Gets in front of me. Looks up and smiles.

"I'm likin' de look o' de look," she informs her companion who nods as though she requires patronizing.

Then she smiles at me. "Tanks a mill," she says.

They walk out of the shop. They didn't buy anything. Next day, and for the rest of the week, there's old women everywhere.

The world is awash with magic.

There's a 'but'…

OLD MEN IN RED DRESSES

It seems more to the point that cardinals wear the color scarlet, not us. Not really. Of course the concept of a hymen's importance never ceases to amaze me. That a man, on initial penetration, wants to see blood. Does that not freak you out just a tad? That due to the custom some women and girls, who have been raped, enjoyed sex as much as anyone else, or rode a horse bareback, has to take a secret razor with her on her wedding night and cut herself near her own genitals to bleed for a family's pleasure? To ascertain she is not *ruined* or *spoilt*, like fruit that has fallen from a tree? That women will pay a plastic or cosmetic surgeon to make them a 'new' hymen under general anesthetic (I checked, for this article) and that a qualified medical practitioner will actually agree to this? To designer a vagina? Is there something in this picture that does not ring true?

And to add to the wackiness of a term like "scarlet woman" is the almost-opposite exclamation regarding young men or adolescent males who are supposed to "sow their wild oats" before they get trapped by the "ball and chain". Who are these wild-oat-sewing lads supposed to be having sex with? And, as a matter of clarity, I am speechless at the knowledge of circumcision of any kind, for any gender. And I also kind of like the idea of the labia-pulling tradition in Uganda.

COLA, CHIMNEYS AND CHOCOLATE

Oh, and santa clause? I must not forget the obese elderly man—a stranger in red—who sneaks into children's rooms with unrequested offerings, and sugary lollies, leaving his stoned reindeer straddling your roof. And that society is okay about that.

I'll stop now. This chapter is actually all about menstruation, labor, mothering and menopause, and whether or not there is a male god who set us up and continues to get his rocks off at his own joke. At the expense of half the population of human animals.

Let's begin by deconstructing—or unpacking, as the recent zeitgeist of the twenty-first century puts it—the blood cycles of a woman's life.

TABOO IS TAPU

taboo
Origin

TONGAN

tabu
set apart,
forbidden

taboo
ENGLISH   late 18th century

Late 18th century: from Tongan tabu, *' set apart, forbidden'; introduced into English by Captain James Cook. Also,* tapu *Māori*

Cap'n Jimmy Cookie sails into the safe harbor of an indigenous people's ancestral landscape, drops anchor and rows ashore with a contingent of essentially gun-toting bullies who are as horny and arrogant as they are scared of these dark-skinned, tattooed strangers watching as they come ashore. Initially he and his sailor buddies are welcomed. If they hadn't been this chapter might be titled something else.

He is invited to the longhouse and fed. He is sung to. Danced to in a language of bodies that he does not understand. Appreciated for the impressive ship. All seafaring men like to admire each other's array, don't they? He is in the company of Joseph Banks, who eventually acquires a knighthood and has a plant named for him. What do these lads get up to in the very unchristian and under-dressed Pacific tribal lands? Whatever they can get away with. All things. And an arrogant monarchy out to rape, snatch and grab themselves as many resources from as many others as they can get away with without a good spearing, cannibalism or zombification. Well, that last actually happens, but that's not for here. Wade Davis[14] can offer an explanation.

The point of this is not simply the fact of planting the 'butcher's apron[15]' on foreign soil and proceeding to wreck the customs, language, spirituality and joy of as many strangers as they could but also to claim whatever they wanted. One of those claims is the word nowadays called taboo.

---

[14] https://harpers.org/archive/1984/04/the-pharmacology-of-zombies/
[15] https://ansionnachfionn.com/2012/06/21/the-butchers-apron-britains-war-in-ireland/

Taboo didn't mean, then, what it means today. There are places and times of year when intelligent humans know to avoid certain proximities. It's beneficial to all in the equation.

AOTEAROA AND EELS

Eels migrate up streams as elvers to find suitable adult habitat. After many years (15-30 years for shortfins, 25 years for longfins, and sometimes up to 80 years) they migrate to the Pacific Ocean to breed and die. Eels are secretive, mainly nocturnal and prefer habitats with plenty of cover. The ancestors of modern Aotearoa (New Zealand) eels (like *Anguilla dieffenbachii*) have swum up and down the waterways since at least the early Miocene (23 million years ago).

Tuna – ā tātou taonga. Tuna (the Māori word for eels) are not only historically important to Māori, they are *taonga* today. But pressure on some species is resulting in their decline. Do they rest in shallow waters to the side of rivers? Of course. Are they trapped or speared while they rest? Indigenous peoples are the least stupid of us all.

They know when to hunt. They are not about to slaughter eel stocks while in certain stages of their lifecycle as that would eventually decimate the species as a food source. They have been taught the significance of certain places. Just don't go there. Eat berries. Or wrestle a crocodile. Drink cassava, eat some macerated yams. You get the idea.

This is the first thing to consider, in this chapter on menstruation and menopause ++

ORIGINS OF MENSTRUATION AS 'UNCLEAN'

While the understanding of what taboo really means is supposed to jolt even myself out of the shame placed upon me, our daughters and our granddaughters—not to mention our mothers and theirs and theirs, our son's, brother's father's misunderstanding of woman-anatomy—it is also advisable to hypothesize on how and why woman-bleeding should be considered by so many religions and ideologies as unclean. If you're in the mood, may I suggest you *google* around a bit on this subject? Likely as not you'll discover menstruation is considered most powerful and revered by indigenous humans who have not been inculcated into the deplorable humiliation of religions. So what happened?

THE CURSE AND DONALD TRUMP

Humans—or, rather, hominidae—are a branch of the great ape family tree. Primates. We are mammals. What are we? Mammals. Worldwide, the female of every species of mammal occasionally and regularly, experiences estrus. That means we're on 'heat'. We project a scent for six kilometers or more in all directions. Every male within range of our aroma will kill to be top dog, bull, buck, ram, boar; add your own identifier.

When did we, as a human mammal, divide ourselves into two distinctly separate conditions as menstruation and ovulation? I am thankful for many rainy afternoon discussions about this with friends, on the veranda, drinking tea. The theory implies—

Women who live in close proximity to each other menstruate at the same time. If you did not know this, please set up your own discussion group and experiment over a year or so. What can be agreed upon within this exploration of feminine bloodletting is that when it occurs amongst other mammals all thought of hunting vanishes. And, I could conjecture on the term *bloodlust*, but I won't. Not yet and not here. The alpha woman of the tribe says, fuck this, and determines to move all the bleeding women away from the *olfactoriness* (I claim the right to make up words, just like Willy Shakespeare did) of males and into the equivalent of what is called the Red Tent[16]. We removed ourselves from their questing and often violent dicks, in other words. So that we wouldn't starve, and the branch of homo sapiens sapiens (us) potentially continues for future generations.

What does this do hypothetically, to the fellas? Pisses them off, is what. What is one very common theme of pissed off men? They deride. Insult. Make their hurt feeling someone else's fault. Go to war with, or dismiss the other as inferior. Women become the problem. At some dawn of unrecorded history, we also become the enemy. And, as such, we need to be confined, controlled, given rules of behavior and be banned from touching anything in case we poll-

---

[16]https://s3.wp.wsu.edu/uploads/sites/998/2018/04/VictoriaKaralunRedTentReleva nceToToday.pdf

ute it, wither the crops and dry up the udders of cows.

I could be considered facetious but I'm not. Menstruation is also called THE CURSE.

> "...*you could see there was blood coming out of her eyes, blood coming out of her wherever.*" —U.S. presidential candidate, Donald Trump, commenting on hard-hitting questioning by journalist Megyn Kelly (Beckwith 2015)

"The day after a challenging U.S. presidential debate, then-candidate Donald Trump complained about a female journalist's tough questions by appealing to biological reductionism. His seemingly ambiguous reference to 'her wherever' clearly intended to signify 'vagina'—thereby evoking menstrual blood, and its presumed adverse effects.

"In appealing to menstrual blood as the go-to explanation for a female journalist's emphatic interviewing style, Trump revealed that he (like many others) views women as different from men in two crucial ways: ruled by their biology, and naturally meek. If women behave assertively—in ways widely admired for men but disparaged for women—their supposedly out-of-character behavior must be dictated by something beyond their control. Donald Trump signaled that menstrual taboos remain alive and well in the contemporary world."

And—

"…many biblical commentators throughout history have viewed the Levitical menstrual prohibitions as divine punishment for the sinful nature of woman, which, through the actions of Eve, effected the fall of humankind. Menstruation becomes the divine "curse" of women. 17"

I mean, PLEASE. A *curse*? Witches *know* what a curse is, and it's NOT menstruation. We have reasons. There is logic to certain processes. The term for menstruation being relative to hexing is not logical. It is disturbing.

The *Oxford English Dictionary* defines a curse as: "1a. An utterance consigning, or supposed or intended to consign, (a person or thing) to spiritual and temporal evil, the vengeance of the deity, the blasting of malignant fate, etc. It may be uttered by the deity, or by persons supposed to speak in his [*sic*] name, or to be listened to by him [*sic*]." This definition signals that certain unfortunate events presumably emanate from spiritual entities. A later definition further highlights the notion of divine punishment: "4a. The evil inflicted by divine (or supernatural) power in response to an imprecation, or in the way of retributive punishment." I suggest we, as a society, get pissed off about this. Women pay luxury tax on tampons. We have been sold sprays so our genitalia do not smell of fish.

We have been extolled to be too embarrassed to discuss this except

---

[17] Full, fabulous article: https://www.ncbi.nlm.nih.gov/books/NBK565616/#

in private, and even then with caution. This means that we will still bear the wounds of an idiotic hegemony that does not respect one half of an entire mammalian species. I'm done with that. I spoke with a woman earlier today who is 'suffering'. Menopause. Why? Why do we 'suffer'? In this book I have mentioned progesterone deficiency but what's with all the devices? The IUD—a T-shaped piece of hormonally embedded plastic that is wedged in a woman's cervix (progestin; a carcinogen), a contraceptive implant the size of a matchstick that is injected into the soft bit of our upper arms (progestogen; a carcinogen) that makes women crazy and piles on the kilos, the contraceptive pill (ditto crazy. Or cancer. Progestin; a carcinogen).

LIFE

The invasion of tube tying or cutting. Hysterectomy. The *Morning After* pill: EVC (evonorgestrel emergency contraceptive) or a UPA[18]. Women, and even girls, are advised to take a vaccine for HPV (human papilloma virus) that is, in truth, sexually transmitted from a penis, and also, as I write, abortion is being scrutinized—ripped from law—by good old boys with desires to control the reproductive rights of women and girls.

Erasure of unsanctioned sex. A punishable crime? Yes, we should be worried.

The point is, I have met and worked with thousands of women over the past forty-something years and not one wants a pregnancy unless she wants a pregnancy. Trials of a male contraceptive other than pulling out or using a condom (highly recommended, by the way, for abundant reasons, like the transmission of herpes for one) have been abandoned because the men involved didn't like some of the side effects such as mood swings, acne, depression, weight gain. Um...............

MENOPAUSE

Regarding the cessation of menstruation and the ability to breed someone thought of the ridiculous word menopause. It is not a

---

[18] https://medlineplus.gov/druginfo/meds/a610020.html: *If you vomit less than 3 hours after you take ulipristal, call your doctor. You may need to take another dose of this medication.*

pause. It is a sweaty, dry-vagina'd moody, mentally challenging, depressing, breathless, weight-gaining attempt to have us all agree, once again (or still), that there is a male god, and that he hates women. Like PMS (pre-menstrual shittiness) and post-natal depression that isn't depression at all but is a woman realizing, even as the oxytocin kicks in, that her freedom and life as a sexy, lusty, erotic, sensual, hoodoo hussy is compromised by both the infant's demands for EVERYTHING to the partner's desire for perkier breasts and a non-flabby belly that is pumping up the plastic surgery industry to the tune of almost $15 billion dollars.

This is speculation, I guess, but being a woman with countless women before me, all of whom—eternally—existed in my own eggs when I still had them, I have often wondered whether menopause would be such a trauma if we had not been a species that, through the necessity of the survival of our hominid family and descendants, cleverly evolved to separate ovulation from menstruation. Is menopause an attempt to bring the two back into one? Like forest-bathing. And thus wondering, by the way, about men with red buttons at their fingertips.

CHILDBIRTH

We begin menstruation somewhere between the ages of 8 and 18 (generally) and the cramps can cripple us for days out of a month. We can suffer endometriosis. No cure. Sore and tender breasts. No cure. PCOS. "Go on the pill," says doc 1. "Have a baby," says doc 2. I was once upon a time, as a suicidal teenager, informed I suffered a hysterical personality because my rage at injustice was so intense and incurable I had turned it in on myself (hence the word depression, like an avalanche going back up the mountain because it has worked out that freefalling, true to its nature, is pointless).

Childbirth is like shitting bricks. And once upon a time, in total illogic and against all gravitational mathematics, we were made to lie on our backs, our feet in stirrups, our perineum sliced with a scalpel because it's a ridge of muscle that interferes with the masked staff, given an enema so we don't poo the sheets and even informed that canned formula was trendier than breast feeding. And that breast feeding in public was—and often still is—disgusting and aimed at tempting some satanic urge into a bloke's loins when he sees it.

Either that or he's batshit jealous that the kid's on the nipple and not him. Then we are stitched up. THEN our milk comes in anyway. Agony. Porcupines where pleasure used to be. That's as much a surprise as going into labor after the infant is born because our placentas want the same exit, requiring a form of peristalsis.

I don't care. This chapter is not intended to be rational. I had the irrational pleasure of discussing menopause today with that suicidal woman. Well, not so much suicidal as able to recognize the pointlessness of life once menstruation, and bleeding into a pad, a tampon, a moon cup or moss, has stopped.

PELVIC FLOOR AND KEGELS

kegel

/'keɪgl/

noun

Denoting exercises performed by a woman to strengthen the pelvic floor muscles, involving repetitions of both sustained and rapid voluntary contractions of the muscles and used, especially, to treat urinary incontinence and improve sexual function. "She recommends women do Kegel exercises two to three times a day"

Most women forget the Kegels. When I train either women or men I advise them both to suck up their pelvic floor muscles. For women post-childbirth this is imperative. I also maintain that scrotal herniation and possibly even prostate disorders can be cause by constant pressure on the pelvic muscles. So suck it up, people. Suck. It. Up. For women the consequences of NOT doing so can be dire. Your uterus can prolapse. Hang down through your cervix into your vagina. Painful. Incontinence. Embarrassing. The recent class action in Australia, against Johnson and Johnson's pelvic mesh implants, gained women $300 million in payouts for those affected by life-sentences of pain and trauma. Lots of money to be earned for shonky products made by corporations at the expense of quality of life. Be warned.

TAPU AND US

You are tapu. I am tapu. We are the treasure that is to be revered and tended. We are the mothers of Earth, whether we birth children or simply walk down Swanston Street with our heads held high. At no stage will we allow some righteous con-artist try to tell us that we are not magnificent. Can we embrace our hair going grey or white? It does not diminish us. The poison—the PPD[19]—in all hair products will. Or can. So will eyelash and eyebrow dye. And a woman never knows when or if. There are no huge warnings. There is wincy little writing on the side of a packet of the poison (and yes, I died my hair most of my life until the PPD allergy struck like head lice on steroids). Can PPD allergic reaction cross over and trigger allergic reactions to everything? Yes. Does the patch test always work? No. And how many reading this actually do it? Yes, I see the absolute lack of hands in the air.

This concludes my rant concerning taboos, secret cabals of capitalist consumerism at our expense, the ex-prime ministers of this country knocking back a beer in Hawaii while Cobargo burns, on the money he gained from the luxury tax on what are deemed 'women's hygiene or sanitary products', our mammalian urge to squat while giving birth, sometimes secretly because hey, isn't that a bit crude? And our absolute denial of being unclean.

...

---

[19] Paraphenylenediamine

Dear Diary,

The cruelest thing anybody ever said, or did, to me is... (add whether
this defines you still)

ESTABLISHING RELATIONSHIP WITH EARTH

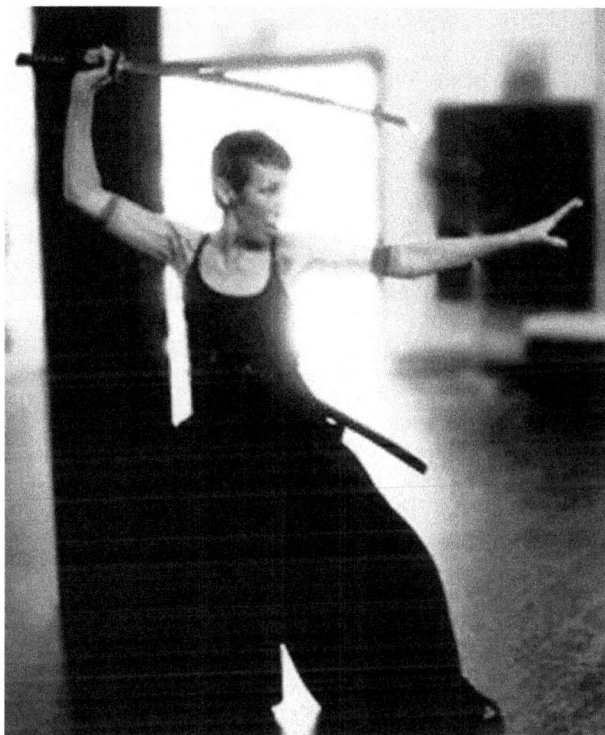

de Angeles (short hair = PPD allergy) Iaido training

There would be no point healing, training and maintaining a vital body if the way we thought, viewed life and processed experiences was confused. People are manipulated and assaulted from every direction by jargon and implication – mostly repetition, mostly rhetoric – and that's putting it mildly.

Once upon a time I attended *kumijo* class, at the Aikido Centre in Byron Bay, where I trained with both staff and bokken. At the close of the evening we students all sat on the mats, while Sid, who took the class because Michael sensei was overseas, gave us what he presumed to be a wisdom lesson.

He said that the subconscious is white and positive, and that if we have negative thoughts – black – they go into the subconscious and turn it grey. What a disappointing discussion. Dualisms like good/bad, black/white, positive/negative merely reinforce the stereotypical paradigms that have become a religious and political tool, as well as a major advertising ploy, to attempt to manipulate us into a specific ideology of acceptability. To evoke guilt, and the threat of punishment that bucking an agreed-upon agenda will bring down upon those who oppose the ploy. Seemed like this has been an excuse, for slavery, forever. These concepts are constructs. They are without any substance in sparrow or wolf or kangaroo language.

So, what's the reality?

The dissolution of androcentric brainwashing. Absolution from thinking *humanly*, to the denial of us as a carbon-based life form like any other.

WATERFALL WATERFALL, TEACH ME HOW

Not far from where I live there is a place called Protestors Falls. At the end of a track that meanders through the rainforest is a deep pool fed from a waterfall that cascades down a two hundred and forty-foot escarpment. It can be quite loud there beside the pool, sitting upon boulders that embrace it, because this is a natural amphitheater. Bat caves dot the cliff face; ferns and native plants defy gravity from rocky outcroppings.

Sitting there a person can look up towards the top of the falls. The experience is akin to reverse vertigo. The sky sits on top of it all in such a vivid blue as to hurt the eyes. Birds whip-call across the valley. I've been at the waterfall as dusk turned to night, and the profusion of fireflies warped the senses in the darkness, as they flickered between huge trees and land on my eyelashes. The place is like somewhere set apart. One can get lost in its wonder.

The waterfall, thunders or trickles, depending on the season, into the deep pool at its base, it murmurs and tumbles down and down, over rock and rock and rock, linking with other creeks and waterways until it reaches the sea. Of course. The water from the falls comes from elsewhere. From unseen gorges and gullies, catchments for rain and spring-fed creeks much, much higher up the mountainside. But along the journey of its destiny are habitats. That'd be frogs. Lizards. Birds and snakes, padymelons, echidna, wallabies, turtles and, so I have been assured, platypus. They have lived around or in the waters of this place since the Dreamtime[20].

Sometimes tour buses bring people here. And isn't it nice to take a

---

[20]https://www.aboriginal-art-australia.com/aboriginal-art-library/aboriginal-dreamtime/

dip in the deep, deep pure waters of the pool at the base of the falls? Tourists have been responsible for the decimation of these habitats; for the poisoning of those waters. They wore deodorant, perfume, sunblock, make-up, hair product; false things; toxic things. If someone had told them to be clean of all these things first would they have taken care to do so? Of course. But once upon a time they were not informed? And to enter the waters aware? There's a no swimming rule on a sign just before the walk. People take no notice and there is no penalty. Is the endangered Fleay's barred frog extinct yet?

The subconscious is not a void, nor is it a mess. It can be a garden or a forest of wild profusion – that depends on the *nature* of us, but each mind is unique and will flourish if it remains unpolluted by ignorance. We must be mindful to prevent that which is toxic, or noxious, or alien, from gaining hold. To do this requires a modicum of detachment. From emotional detachment to material. From agreeing to the jargon. From outside interference that seeks to tell you what is right or wrong, black or white, positive or negative. Tired dualisms. A mind like clear water takes care. And it needs to be left alone sometimes. To be quiet.

Mother Waterfall taught me this: *Kid, stop thinking that way, eh? How about you learn to have a mind just like clear water.*

...

Too

Too old

Too young

Too tired

Too late

Too thin

Too dumb

Too... (add)

...

Dear Diary,

I always thought I was too...

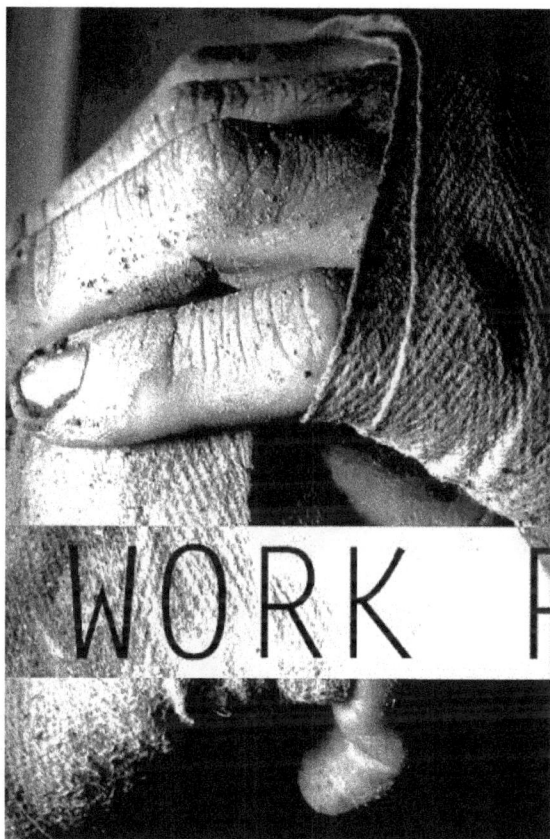

PART TWO

THE PROGRAM, THE PRACTICE

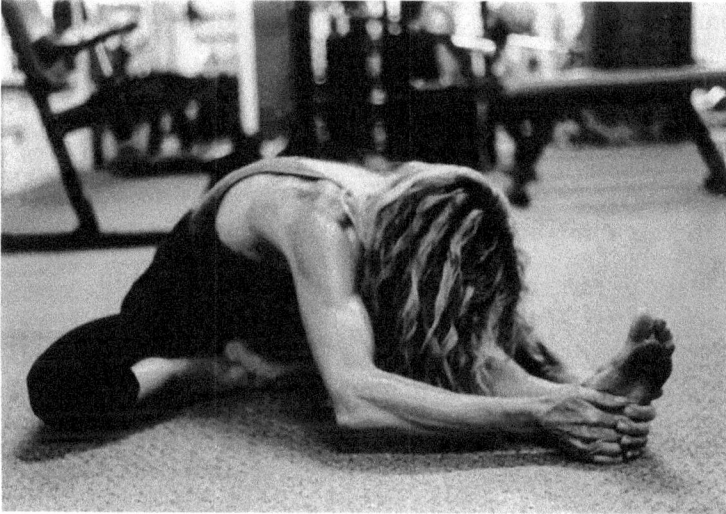

Before you train warm-up: running on the spot for 30 to 60 seconds, skip rope, 4 sets of 10/20 fast reps, do 50 star jumps. Push out 50 crunches, 20 pushups, 20 lunges, 20 squats, 6 minutes on the stationary bike or treadmill. Do high intensity interval training.

STRETCH

When you do a stretch session, relax and breathe into the stretch and don't bounce; never bounce.

ALSO work each side of your body equally. Do the same number of stretches or reps on both sides, evenly and with awareness of differences.

One side of our spines is naturally more passive than the other and together they form a balance. We are as vulnerable as we are strong. We need to know that to live well. Each hand or leg or shoulder serves its purpose in the symphony of physical form.

SCALES ARE FOR DRAGONS

Beginners occasionally say, *Oh, my left side's weak.* Our bodies are responsive to our thoughts as well as being empathic to external stimuli and any can darken our shine. It's social conditioning.

Forgive yourself. Stroke the vulnerable arm. Get a massage. Research acupuncture and PRP just in case.

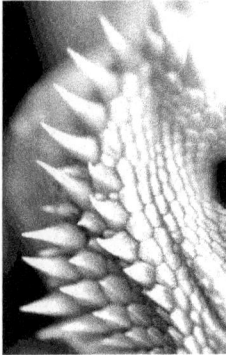

When you begin a healing process, stay with it long enough to realize, or otherwise, the benefits. Chopping and changing all the time, rather than some of the time, will lead to inadequate development, shattered self-esteem and—deeply disagreeable—a sense of shame. Like you lost your wings when you are not a termite.

For a while you will be familiarizing yourself with the weights and exercises, building strength and flexibility of often forgotten, even stagnant parts of yourself. Gathering up your life and banishing what you have, until now, felt powerless to change. You are well along the road to self-determination and healing on so many levels only you will know when you are clear of the way you have lived in the ways of others who are not you, and can never really know you and can never be you. Only you can be that.

METABOLISM

Metabolism is going to alter – to speed up. Fluid and fat levels will realign in accordance with our inherent body types (ectomorph, endomorph or mesomorph). In Ayurvedic medicine these body types are called *vata*, *peta* and *kapha* and many attributes can be researched that I won't cover here. I, however, have a mainly *vata* body with a touch of *kapha*. While the benefits of being *vata* mean I am lean naturally, and fine-boned, it also suggests an anxious temperament, cold hands and feet and a tendency towards insomnia. That final one caused, in my case by hypervigilance from raising three kids in often crazy dysfunctional circumstances. The cutting-edge medical practitioners are prescribing cannabis oil that is mainly CBD (the antipsychotic module) with a touch of THC (the psychotropic module). It took a while but has also radically improved memory and resistance to such oddnesses as the H1N1 viral epidemic's effect.

I mentioned this earlier, but in case you forgot, the weight-scales should be related to like a brown snake, best avoided, respected but dangerous. Muscle is heavier than fat and, initially, you could freak out by thinking you are doing things wrong. You won't be. For a while you will be eliminating fluids and excess body fat, using the latter as an energy source, especially if you decide to go *keto*. The eating regime that excludes all sugars and grains. Also called the Paleolithic diet. A desirable weight won't be valid. When you are stronger, and your musculature is well-defined you will be at your lightest, as well as your heaviest. Balanced.

Note the weights that challenge you at the 11th or 12th rep (and I *mean* challenge) and you'll know that you are working to your optimum because when you attempt another rep you'll fail. This kind of failure is excellent.

...

FALLIBILITY

Am I the only person in the universe
who has to keep on
working out what I want
by discovering what I don't?

...

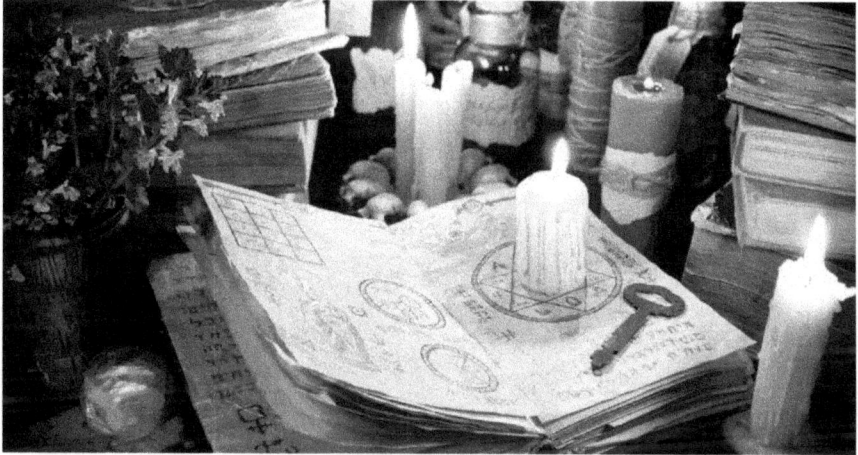

Remember to keep a grimoire of where you're up to so that the next time you train that body-part you will begin without wondering *Ah, what weight did I do last time? How many reps was that? How many sets was I supposed to do?* Once you've worked a specific exercise for a while you will want to add a little variety to the body-part's playtime, so you won't get bored. Bored muscles don't change.

Exercise with a partner if you can. Someone capable of pointing out that you're swinging your back on standing biceps curls; that your form is off on your squats. Someone who will encourage that last rep or two because they know you really want it. A friend who can spot for you and with whom you know you are safe.

SOMEONE WITH A SENSE OF HUMOR.

Dear Diary,

Sometimes I choose not to forgive...

HYDRATION. Consume ample water and/or electrolyte drink during your workouts

NEVER jerk any movement. Use smooth, strong, controlled executions of every exercise

ALWAYS breathe correctly: a. Inhale in preparation for exertion, b. exhale *on* the exertion form. If your form is 'out' then back off the weight or discontinue reps

BENCHES. Contour your body into them so that you are isolating the muscle you are to heal

USE the mirrors. They are not there for the ego, they are an essential tool

RELAX throughout. Exertion and uptightness are not synonymous goals: your natural body-shape, unique to you, realizing that this kind of spellcasting is akin to sculpting, but that genetics will play a part in any eventual milestone

EAT quality protein, fats &/or salad within 20 to 30 minutes (never more than 1 hour, anyway) of your session

PROTEIN heals and assists the body to produce new cells (carbs are fuel only). We all require a minimum of 250 grams per day so that the liver can function properly

KEEP SUPPLE. Always do a warm-up: cardio and /or stretch, yoga, dance, martial arts, pole and circus are all excellent recovery time – receive ample

TAKE pleasure in what you are doing. Chances are that should you come to the stage of saying *Oh, no, not training again,* you are quite likely to have been over-training or boring yourself. RE-EVALUATION will be in order

BE FULLY PRESENT and mindful to avoid injury

HAVE respect for yourself and other serious athletes. Don't be disparaged by the attitude of the few idiots who attend gyms. Most have good 'gym-etiquette'

Be CLEAR. Do this for yourself and not to attract or please others

KEEP your cardio-vascular system toned. Attend boxing classes, or circuit training. It's no good just being able to lift the fallen tree off your friend's broken body if you haven't got the stamina to run for help

DON'T lock-out any of your joints at full extension of a movement and hold your pelvic floor muscles strongly in contraction with each standing pose

BE courageous but not dangerous with yourself. Remember to allow *velvet* into your life and not just *steel*

KEEP a record of your workout and nutritional regime; the exercises, weights, sets, reps, on what days

...

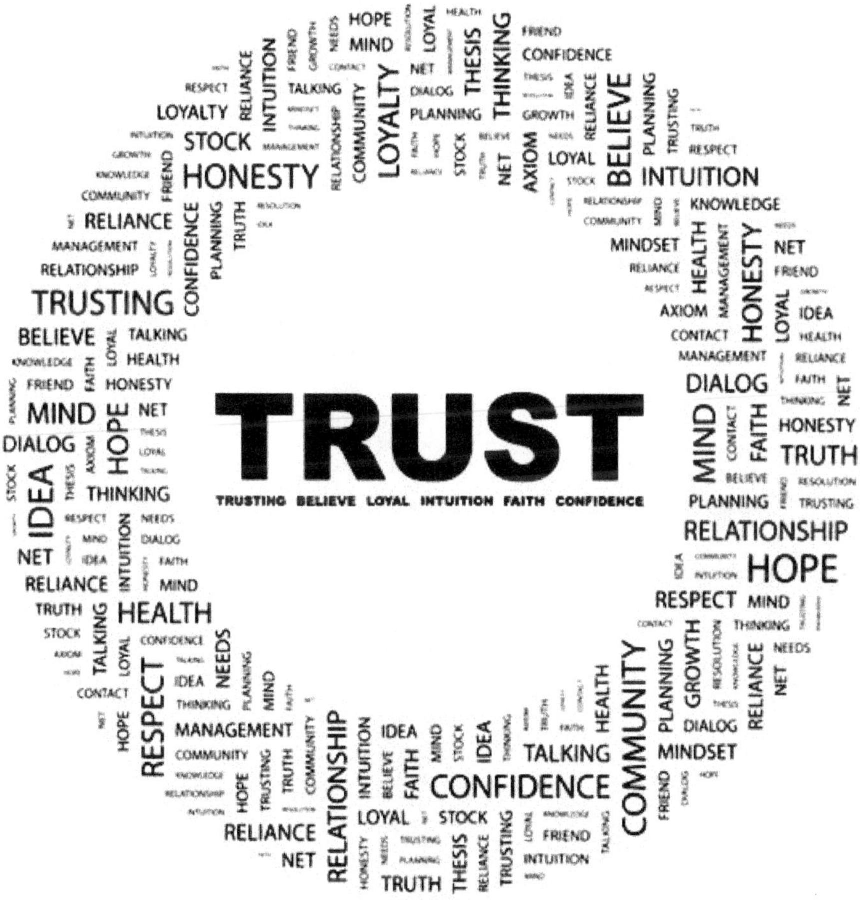
TRUST
TRUSTING BELIEVE LOYAL INTUITION FAITH CONFIDENCE
HONESTY
STOCK
LOYALTY
TRUSTING
RELIANCE
BELIEVE
INTUITION
KNOWLEDGE
MINDSET
RELATIONSHIP
HOPE
RESPECT
HEALTH
IDEA
MIND
DIALOG
CONFIDENCE
COMMUNITY
MANAGEMENT
TALKING
THINKING
TRUTH
NET
FAITH
THESIS
PLANNING
GROWTH
AXIOM
FRIEND
CONTACT

PART THREE

TRAINING SCHEDULE

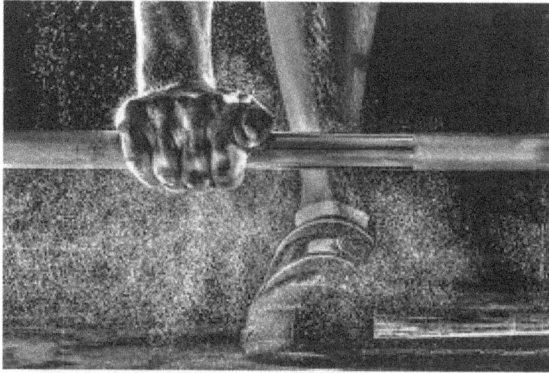

BEFORE YOU FLY

- Familiarize yourself with the gym of your choice
- Do not be daunted or feel insecure when others seem to be where you want to be
- Have your program at hand and record your weights each training session
- Ignore the television if it's a commercial gym. Drives me nuts
- Be calm and slow
- Enjoy failure
- Be prepared to hurt after the first day but not the first month

Dear Diary,

I fucked up, didn't I? No, wait... I'm sick of blaming myself.

Exercise	Sets	Reps	Equipment
Warm up: Wide-grip lat. pulldown	1	15/20	Seated cables, wide-grip curve bar, light weight
Wide-grip lat. pulldown	3	8/12	Seated cables, wide-grip curve bar
Seated rows	3	8/12	Seated cables, close-grip
Bent-over rows	3	8/12	barbell
Single-arm row	3	8/12	dumbbell

BICEPS

Exercise	Sets	Reps	Equipment
Warm up	1	15/20	Light barbell
Standing curls	3	8/12	barbell
Curls with EZ-bar	3	8/12	EZ curl bar/ preacher bench
Concentrated curl	3	8/12	single dumbbell

ABS/OBLIQUES/CORE

50/100 crunches.

Planks, front/sides.

NOTES ON MY BACK—

CHEST

Exercise – –	Sets	Reps –	Equipment –
Warm up	1	15/20	Floor
Dumbbell Fly's	4	8/12	Incline bench, dual arm dumbbells
Flat bench press	3	8/12	Dual arm dumbbells
Incline press	3	8/12	Dual arm dumbbells
Cable fly's	3	8/12	Cable machine, bent over, dual-arm

TRICEPS

Exercise –	Sets –	Reps –	Equipment
Warm up, bent over kickbacks	1	15/20	Bent over dumbbells
Pushdowns	4	8/12	Standing cable machine, triangle bar
Lying triceps extensions	3	8/12	Lying flat bench, EZ-curl bar
Kickbacks	3	12	Bent over dumbbells
Dual arm dips	3	8/12	Assisted dips machine if necessary

ABS/OBLIQUES/CORE

Planks, front and sides. Lying leg-lifts, 20/50

Oblique twists with kettle bell, 20/50. Cable pulldowns

NOTES ON MY CHEST AND TRICEPS—

LEGS

include glutes, quads, hamstrings, calves

Exercise –	Sets –	Reps	Equipment –
Warm up.	1	15	No weight barbell squat
Squats	3	8/12	Weighted barbell
Sumo Deadlifts	3	8/2	Barbell
Straight-legged Deadlifts	3	8/12	Barbell
Walking Lunges	3	8/12	Dual-arm dumbbells
Quad Extensions	3	8/12	Seated extension
Hamstring Curls	3	8/12	Seated or Lying extensions
Standing calf raises	3	12/20	Own bodyweight

HIP FLEXORS/EXTENSORS/ADDUCTORS

Attach either strap to your ankle and work the cables, alternating legs, for 3 x 12 reps, or same with resistance band or Sumo Squats, adductors, Smith Machine, A/B

ABS/OBLIQUES/CORE

Lateral Core: Suitcase Deadlifts, either barbell or single, heavy dumbbell, 12/20
Side Planks from 1 to 3 minutes

NOTES ON MY LEGS/GLUTES—

DAY 4

SHOULDERS/DELTOIDS – anterior, medial and posterior

Exercise –	Sets –	Reps –	Equipment –
Warm up shoulders	1	15/20	Light barbell
Military press	3	8/12	Weighted barbell
Side lateral raises	3	8/12	dumbbells
Front-arm raises (anterior)	3	8/12	1 heavy dumbbell held in both hands
Barrel Fly (posterior)	3	8/12	Standing dumbbells
Face-front rope pull (postural back muscles)	3	12/15	Standing dual arm rope pull at cable machine.

FOREARMS, FLEXORS AND EXTENSORS

Exercise –	Sets –	Reps –	Equipment–
Seated wrist curls	3	12/20	Bench/barbell
Standing reverse curls	3	12/20	Standing/barbell

ABS/OBLIQUUS/CORE: MORE

Hanging leg raise (to failure) from the pull up bar, or straight-armed from the assisted dips bar (can do this with weight between the knees

NOTES ON MY SHOULDERS AND FOREARMS—

COMMON TERMS

The above is an example program only. You can work 2 days on, 2 off or 3 on 1 off, or 4 days straight, then take 3 days off for recovery. The weight is not included here as that is a matter to be worked out individually. The best thing for you to do, when you first join a gym is feel okay about your right to be there.

Second thing is to consult one of the trainers, or an elder, and have them go over the exercises with you until you are familiar. Be careful who you choose – a learned person should work with you every step of the way until you can do the exercises with precision.

TECHNICALITY

We'll cover a few muscles, and muscle groups, that you will be working, their exercises ad equipment. Take the time to go over this until you are savvy. I also recommend you pick up some good bodybuilding magazines from a news agency, for the first few months, as they often have hot tips. Some YouTube tutorials, also. But be wary if they want your money. You are their goldmine.

You'll probably figure out that most of the articles do a repeat round, with different faces, but it's the little side pieces that provide extra information. Some of the photo sessions can be a real turn-off.

Don't let it get to you.

COMMON TERM NOTES—

There's what I know and what I think I know
And the two don't know how to get along.
One thing I know is that I— I—
Will be food for beetles, worms and microorganisms
No matter how much of what I think
I know gets piled on top of that bit of fact.

Unless I get zapped—annihilated—by the magnetic field of a
passing (random or otherwise) alien particle accelerator.

No matter what I know or what I think I know, I won't know until I
do.

What I *think* I know is studied furiously,
Is questioned at every juncture for its wisdom,
Is researched for all available expert opinion
And, finally, is allocated its importance;
Its greatness.
This is what I do. And then I rest.
But then this 'greatness' is attacked, by what I know,
And called belief; a speculation. I defend it well. For a while

My secret is that, like a teenager being spoken down to, by a know-
it-all teacher... I *know* I don't know everything.

Dear Diary,

I was lied to about (write a list)

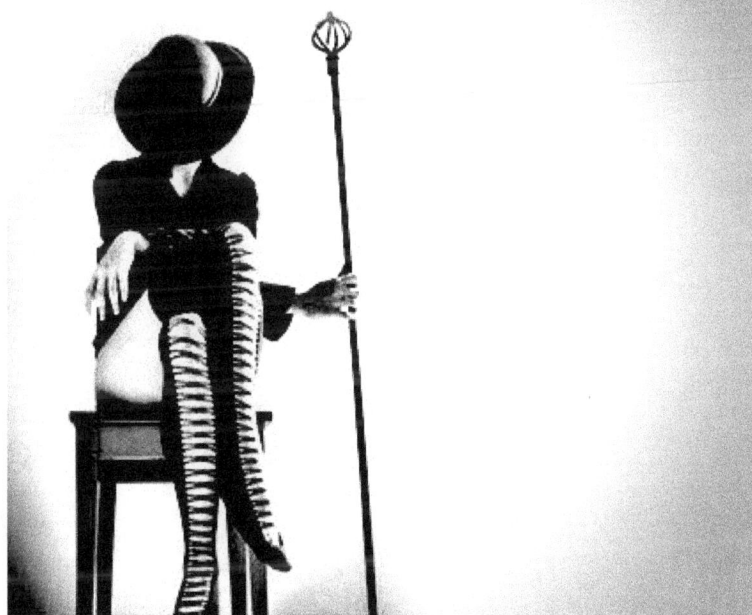

Bitchcraft:
The art of pissing people off
by telling them the truth.

CHEST – PECTORALS

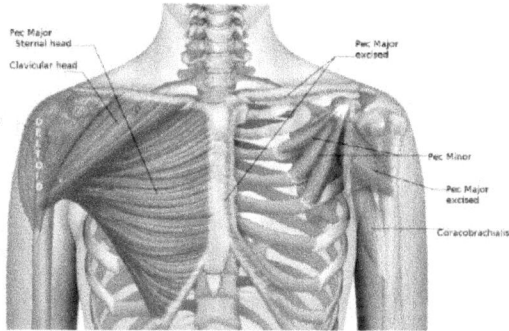

pecs, the large chest muscles

Flat-bench press—Barbell or dumbbells. A deepening and strengthening exercise: your entire pectoral.

Incline-bench press—Use dumbbells. Hits your upper pecs and has an influence on your anterior deltoid.

Decline-bench press—Use either barbell or dumbbells. Works your lower pecs.

Fly's—Flat bench, incline and decline. Focuses mainly on your outer pectorals.

Dual arm cable fly's—Gives muscle striation; this exercise, again, targets your outer pectorals.

Push-ups—Wide-hand or close-hand. It takes most women a while to get this, therefore do a few in your warm-up routine every day. Begin on your knees and progress to straight-bodied push-ups. I do them on my knuckles as my wrists are stressed from damage done decades ago, punching a bag.

Pec deck—Work this for variety later. I'd recommend the dumbbell press as this is really targeting overall pectoral musculature.

...

Including the scapula, rhomboid, trapezius and infraspinatus

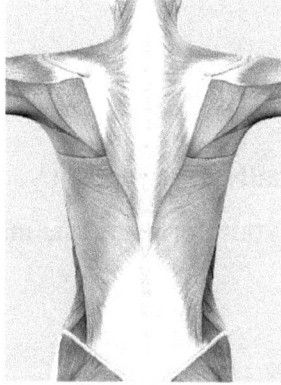

called lats: upper, mid and lower back

Pull-ups—The ultimate back exercise; both close-grip and wide-grip, forward or reverse grip. Builds strength but, initially, can be very difficult for women, especially as a beginner. I suggest that you work with a spotter. Have your knees bent and have the spotter support you lightly under the knees - even if it's just with one hand, to assist you to build confidence.

Wide-grip, in-front-of-the-neck lat pull-downs—At a pulley machine, using a curve bar. You may see some people do this exercise behind the neck – experience has shown that this can place unnecessary stress on the shoulder joints.

Seated rows—Use a close grip, to hit your rhomboid and lower down your lat.

Bent-over rows—Targets your lower lats and into your lower back – use either an EZ curl or a straight bar. You might need to use a back-support belt.

BENT-LEGGED DEAD-LIFTS, OR SUMO DEADLIFTS—

This exercise is specifically to strengthen your lower back and core. Use a barbell. Watch your form (again, maybe that back-support belt).

Bent-over, alternating single-arm rows—For your medial-lat.

...

QUADRICEPS and GLUTEUS (glutes)

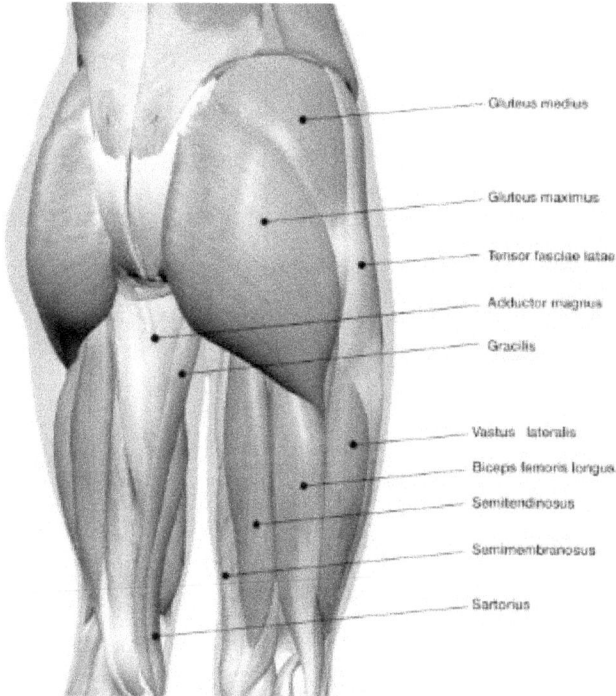

Gluteus medius
Gluteus maximus
Tensor fasciae latae
Adductor magnus
Gracilis
Vastus lateralis
Biceps femoris longus
Semitendinosus
Semimembranosus
Sartorius

thigh and bum muscles

Squat (the SUPREME leg exercise)—*Including the Sumo Squat*— Use a barbell. Do the exercise with perfect form to avoid hurting yourself, especially your knees. The Sumo squat will work your adductor (inner thigh) muscles, your glutes and, to a degree, your hamstrings.

Lunges—Use either a bar on the shoulders (weights on the bar come later) or a pair of dumbbells. Do either alternating legs or single leg. This exercise will have you feeling like a mule kicked your butt for the first few times. Don't do if you have knee problems.

Seated leg extensions—Target your quad heads, adding definition to strength.

Incline leg press (Lying)—I prefer the squat as it targets more leg mass, however this exercise is of benefit to you, as a beginner, and anyone with lower back problems. Keep your feet straight ahead, to access a 'squat-like' affect. Point your toes slightly out to target your adductors. Toes only, on the board, will work your calves.

GLUTES

Hip thrusts (bench)—start out with a barbell only. Face to the ceiling, have your shoulders and neck supported on a bench, your legs bent at the knee, the barbell across your lap. In sets of 12 raise and lower your bum to the floor then the ceiling, squeezing your glutes together on the exertion.

...

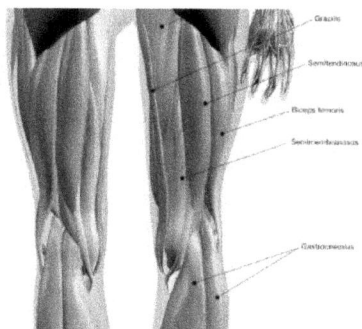

back of your upper leg, bum to knee

Lying/Seated hamstring curl—Stick to light weights and protect your knees.

Dead-lifts—Stand on a slight platform for maximum extension. Use a barbell BUT don't overdo it! You can pull a lot of weight with this exercise and think that it's okay, but you'll be sorry the next day (a back-support belt may be required).

Bent-legged deadlifts—Good idea to wear a lumbar support belt for these. Similar to a clean-and-jerk but you won't lift the bar. You won't bend your elbows. You'll kick your bum out as your reach for the floor-bound rack of weights, roll the bar up your forelegs until you are upright, at which time your knees should be just off locked. Then roll the bar down again to the floor. Don't' forget to power through the breath.

CALVES

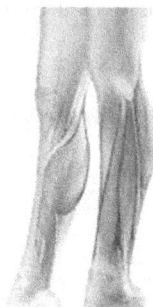

back of your lower leg from knee to ankle

Standing Calf Raises—No problems, but, again, don't go doing double your body-weight or anything just because you can, or you risk either/both crushing the nerves on the ball of your foot or dislodging the vertebrae (done both).

Seated Calf-Raises—Not all gyms have this equipment.

ADDUCTORS

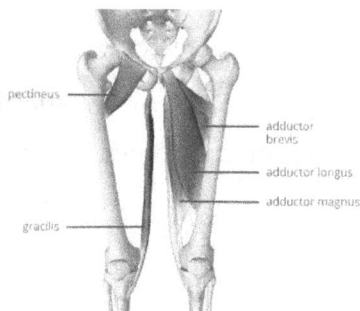

inner thigh

Cable leg-pulls—Use the lower cable, to which is attached an ankle strap, which you will connect to the leg closest to the machine. It is preferable that you stand on a 'step' box. Hold onto the upright of the cable machine, keep your legs a distance apart and swing the leg with the strap on it over towards the front of your other leg. Do a set and change sides (for 3 or 4 sets). Don't go into too heavy or you'll damage the ligaments on the inside of your knees.

HIP FLEXORS

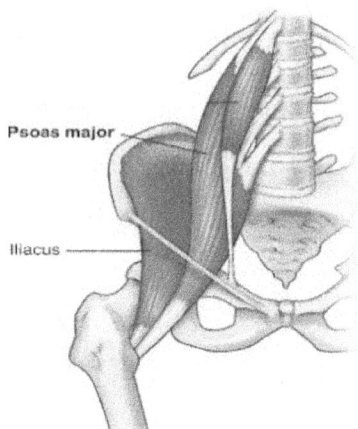

outer thigh/hip

Cable side-kicks—Attach a cable to your outside leg, with a leg strap, or use a resistance band, and swing your leg straight from the hip, to as high as you can comfortably allow (45 degrees to 90 degrees). 1 set of 12, then change legs (repeat 3 sets).

...

Deltoid Medial or Lateral

Rear Deltoid

Front Deltoid

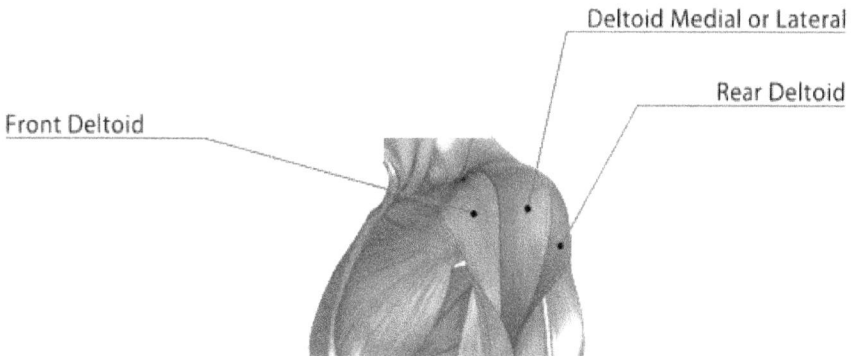

anterior, medial, posterior—front, middle, rear

Military press—Strength and mass. In front of your neck barbell raises (keep your hands well-spaced on the bar. Work with a spotter for maximum gains.

Shoulder press—This has basically the same effect as a Military press, but you'll be using dumbbells as it can make it less stressful on your wrists.

Side lateral raises—I love this exercise (but, then I really dig the shoulder workouts because I love having chunky shoulders). Sometimes called *teapots* because when you lift your arms out to the sides (not quite horizontal). Let your shoulders lead and not your forearms, as you twist your hands towards the end of the movement like pouring out tea or water from a jug. The pinky finger on each dumbbell leads. The form is explicit, and it gives definition, to your muscles.

Posterior deltoids—Also called *barrel fly's*. Use bent-over, dual-arm, side-lateral raise on either the cables or with a dumbbell. With the latter, the best gains occur by rolling a towel into a pillow and resting it on the back of an incline bench, feet back away, your back as straight as you can get it, bent from the hip.

Anterior deltoids—Dual arm dumbbell raises (to forehead height – use the mirror).

...

Trapezius
Stabilizes, raises and
rotates the scapula

Rhomboid minor
Pulls scapula backward

Supraspinatus
Stabilizes
shoulder joint
and raises arm
away from body

Humerus
Long bone
of upper arm

Spine of scapula

Teres minor
Holds humerus
in glenoid cavity

Infraspinatus
Holds humerus
in glenoid cavity

Infraspinatus
Holds humerus in
glenoid cavity, rotates
humerus laterally, as
in a backhand stroke
in tennis

Rhomboid major
Acts with rhomboid
minor to pull
scapula backward

Source: The Atlas of the Human Body, Abrahams P. (2006)

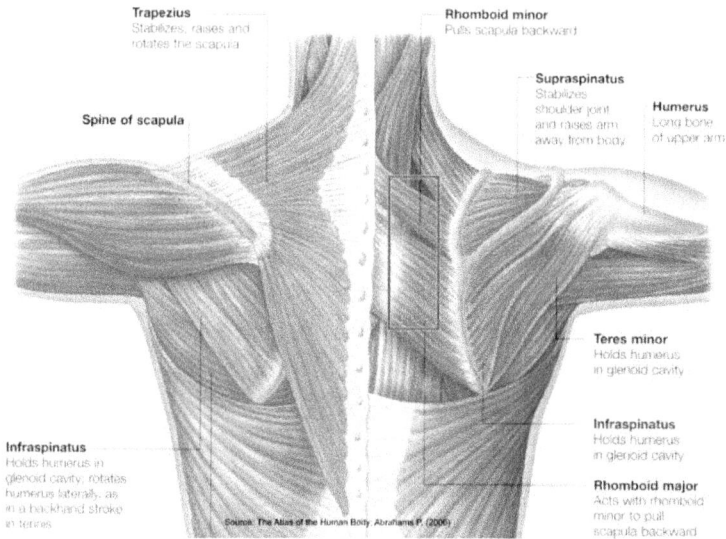

neck to shoulder & a bit down the central spine

Upright row—Use a barbell. Keep your hands close together, palm down, and bring the bar to just under your chin. Don't lock your elbows when you lower the bar.

Shrug—Keep your arms straight and use either the press on the smith machine, or a pair of dumbbells.

There are several other, more obscure, exercises for shoulders. You can explore them for yourself and play with them later.

...

Notes—

BICEPS BRACHII
Long head
Short head

BRACHIALIS

BRACHIORADIALIS

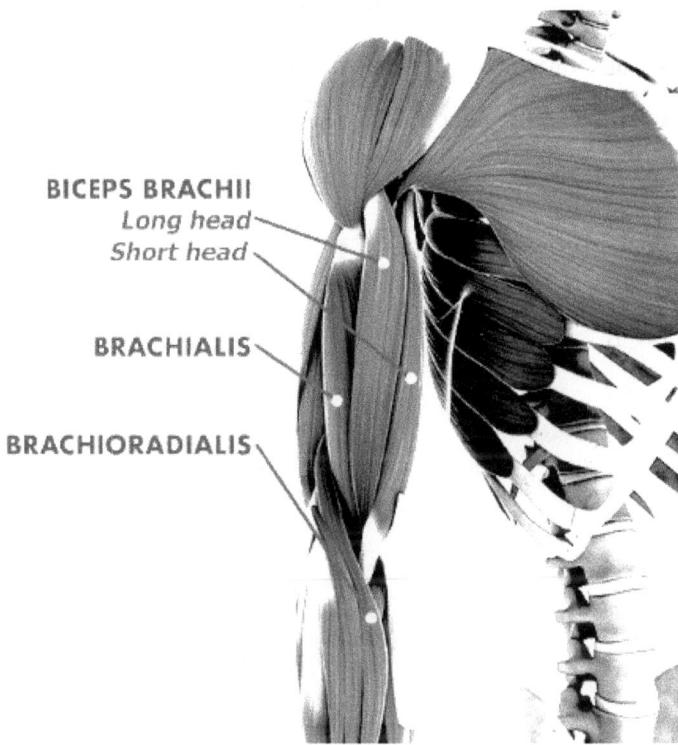

muscles of the upper arm—front

Full biceps curl—Standing barbell curl, Standing EZ curl, close-grip (outer part of the biceps), Standing EZ curl, wide-grip (inner part of the biceps), Standing alternating dumbbell curls.

Preacher bench curls—These are done seated at what's called a *preacher bench*. Either single-arm curls with a dumbbell or both of your hands, close grip, on the inner curl of the EZ curl bar.

Concentrated biceps curls—Seated, single arm dumbbell curls, holding the elbow of your working arm against the inside of the same knee for the exertion. This concentrate focusses mainly on the peak of your bicep. Slow, dual curls, using dumbbells, sitting on a high-backed incline bench, keep your elbows back and don't over-extend when lowering your arms.

...

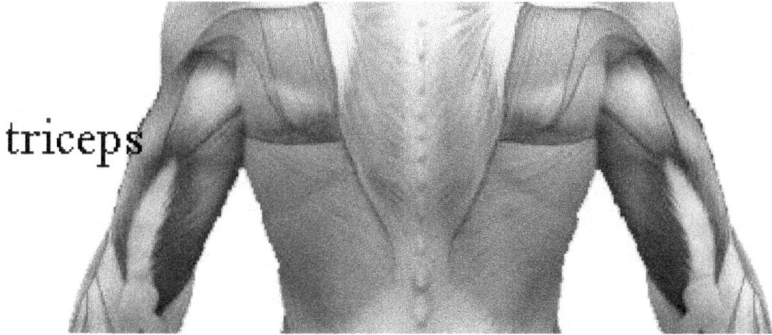

muscles of the upper arm—rear

Pushdowns—Use a triangle bar, or a short, straight bar, at a cable machine or, alternatively, use a double-ended rope pull-down, spreading the rope apart so that your hands are beside your thighs at the completion of the exertion.

Extensions—Flat-bench, lying triceps extension (close-grip). On your back, raise the bar from forehead to straight-armed. Remember: don't lock your elbows and keep them in close to your body, and vertical. Use the EZ curl bar.

Behind-the-neck triceps extension—With dumbbell (either single-arm or dual): extend and lower your arms behind your neck.

Rope pullovers—Performed on the cables, on your knees. With your back horizontal and straight, you pull the rope from behind the head to directly out in front.

Kickbacks—Single or dual arm. With single-arm kickbacks have the knee that's opposite your working arm up on a bench. Keep your back like a table top and extend, from the elbow, backwards, the arm you're working. With dual armed kickbacks adopt a bent-kneed 'skiing' position, back still horizontal, and kick-back with both arms simultaneously.

Dips—At the standing dips bench, or between two flat benches, have your feet together on one bench and the heels of your hands on the other. Lower and raise your body using your arms. Many gyms have assisted-dip machines: the lighter the weight, the more difficult the exercise.

...

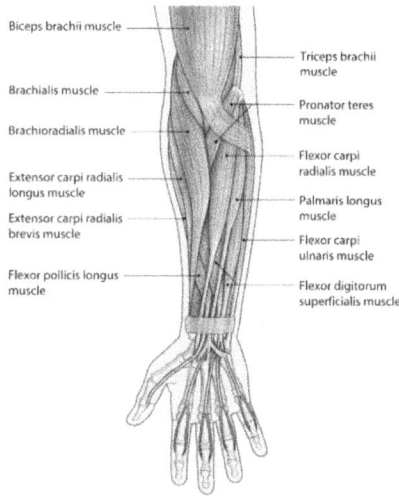

Biceps brachii muscle
Brachialis muscle
Brachioradialis muscle
Extensor carpi radialis longus muscle
Extensor carpi radialis brevis muscle
Flexor pollicis longus muscle

Triceps brachii muscle
Pronator teres muscle
Flexor carpi radialis muscle
Palmaris longus muscle
Flexor carpi ulnaris muscle
Flexor digitorum superficialis muscle

flexors—inner/palm side of the forearm

Seated wrist curls—Seat yourself way back along a bench and hold a barbell in both palms with the wrist just hanging over the edge of the bench. Roll the barbell down your fingers and back up into your palms, squeeze.

extensors—back-of-the-hand side of the forearm

Standing reverse barbell curls—Begin with the barbell in your hands with your palms facing the outside of your thighs. Raise the barbell up slowly, doing a backward wrist flip when you get it all the way up. Flip the bar back over and slowly lower it. Keep the weight to a minimum.

...

NOTES—

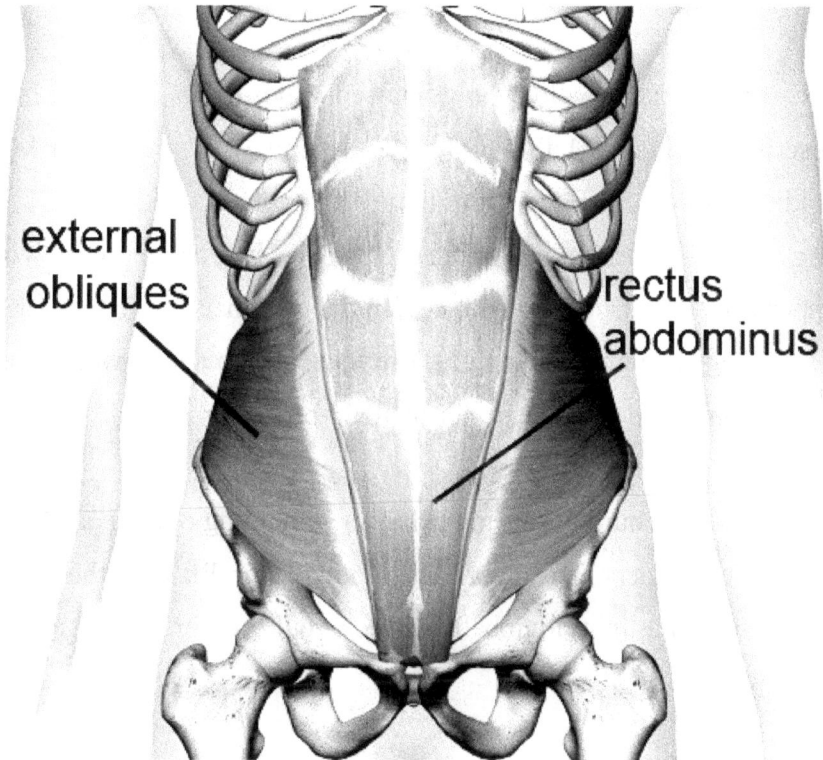

upper belly, lower belly, rib cover, trunk

Crunches (floor or abs bench)—Keep your knees up, feet on the floor, and one hand at each side of your head. Don't support the back of your neck. This exercise will strengthen neck muscles into the bargain but the for will not call on the neck to do the work of the abs. Keep your face to the ceiling. Suck in a breath, contract and hold your abs while doing so, then breathe out forcefully while 'bearing-down' into the abdomen, towards your groin.

Concentrated crunches—Do the above but *much* slower. Control every part of the ascent and descent, keeping your abdominals I contraction the whole time.

9's—Lying on the floor, legs raised, and knees slightly bent, describe the figures 1 through to 9 in the air with your lower legs, holding your abs firm the entire time. 3 to 4 sets.

Leg raises—Either hanging from the pull-ups bar, or supporting your upper body by suspending yourself in the dips machine, either knees bent or legs straight (if you can), lift your legs up and down, as high and as controlled as you can, for up to 25 reps, 2 or 3 sets.

Leg lifts—On your back, arms behind you holding onto an anchored piece of equipment for support, legs up in the air, lift from the glutes. You can hold a light dumbbell between your feet for added gain. 20 to failure.

Planks—Support your body on elbows and toes. Remain horizontal, engaging your core, until failure. These will strengthen your transverse muscles. Good slow count from 20 to failure.

Side Planks—Support yourself on one elbow, lift sideways, keep only elbow and feet on the floor. Everything else is off the ground and straight. Good slow count of from 15 to failure.

Side dumbbell drops— (*Brad Pitt/Fight Club* hip muscles)—I used to hate this look as a younger woman. Now I don't care, so I go for it. Now I love these little sausage muscles that define the lower abdominals between my hips and my quads. Using a single, heavy weight, stand in front of the mirrors to observe your form. Control the dumbbell's slide down one side of your body, into a side crunch.

3 sets of 12 to 20 reps on either side.

OBLIQUES
small muscles under the pectorals and along the ribs,
down past the waist

Side Planks—These are like straight planks, but you perform them on your side, supported on one elbow, one foot atop the other. Keep your free arm pointed towards the ceiling, knees and hips fully off the floor. Hold for the count of 15 to 50 or failure.

Twists with a pole—Look around the gym for the wooden poles. Place it behind your back with your arms along its length. Keeping your knees slightly bent and your pelvic floor muscles engaged, turn from side to side without overextending.

Lying side crunches 1—Lying on your back, knees bent and feet on the floor, reach out with one hand to the outside of your opposing knee. Keep the other hand on the side of your head, which should remain facing the ceiling. 50 or so is good for reps – repeat for the other side.

Lying side-crunches 2—Have both your knees bent and to one side. Have your hands beside your head (facing the ceiling) and attempt to take the elbow, on the side of your knees, in the direction of the opposing hip.

Med Ball Against the Wall—Works at controlling the strength of your core. Pelvic floor muscles contracted and engaged. Starting with your back to the wall, turn and bounce the med ball against the wall and back. Do not allow the return to swing you.

BE AWARE—Any of the abdominal exercises, involving weights, should be VERY LIGHT, else you'll develop predominant abdominals – all very gorilla-like – unless that's an aim. Keeping abdominals engaged and contracted will eliminate the problem.

...

DON'T FRET

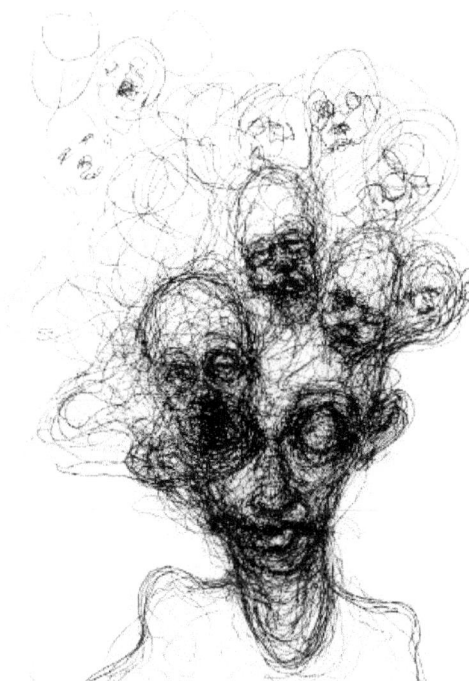

NOT ALL, ALL THE TIME

You don't do all these exercises in a session.

Talk to your trainer or training partner, or get a feel for what works, after several months.

Adjust your program to suit yourself.

...

Dear Diary,

Look at me now!

WE GOT SAVVY

(With Excerpts from *Initiation, A Memoir* 2016)

Women have been haunted by what in legend and lore is the trickster. The trickster is an entity or spirit, puka or sometimes a spirit-that-presents-as-a-man that exists within the myths of almost every culture worldwide. And this beast has sashayed and danced through mythworld, taunting and challenging us for most of our lives. Those of our mothers and those of their mothers deep into the mists of ancestry. Always riding one man's body or another. Just like in the movie *Fallen*.

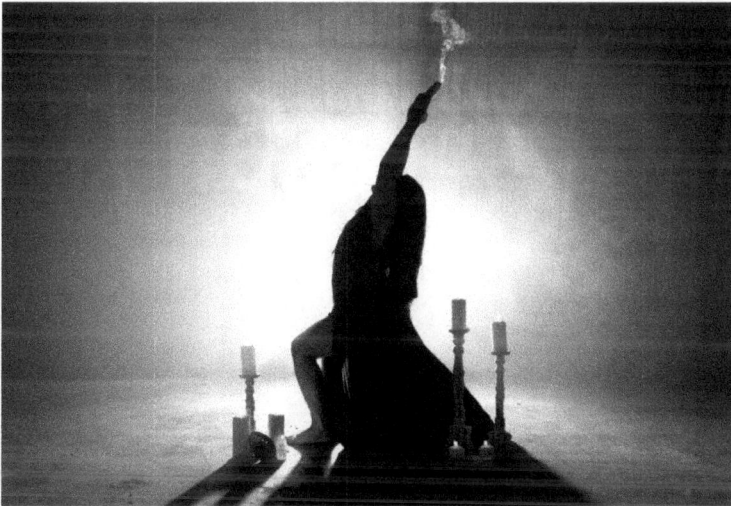

When you don't guess the game, the trickster possesses another man, disrupting your cool and obfuscating your liberty. Originally presenting as benevolent, these people want to control, to own, to direct, even to be protected by you. The trickster seeks an outlet for misbehaviour, stealing power, imposing a culturally-approved order, impoverishing.

The Trickster provides stern lessons. Whether Loki or Crow, Coyote or Puck, Bugs Bunny or Reynard the Fox, Eulenspiegel or Doctor Who, what it wants, ultimately, is what everyone wants. Worthy stories. So that living is an experience of granite strength but feather-light malleability. Of excitation and delight.

So, it keeps on coming but it will eventually learn. You healed. You just kept training. So, the scumbag that the trickster left behind? A try-hard? Checkmate. From this day forth your iron will always be soft.

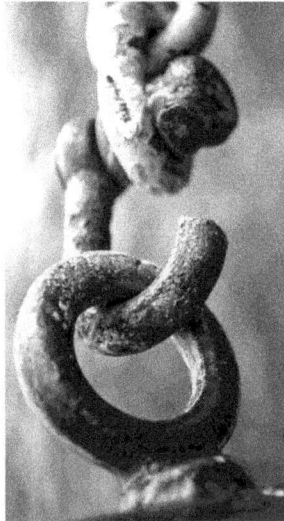

MEDICINE WOMAN SAYS—

WATCHA COOKIN', GOOD LOOKIN'?

When witchery's in the kitchen, and is a-cookin mushroom stew,
just this once allow the aroma to come on up and summon you
because this life can seem so empty when the magic's cast aside
but it's here, within the shadows, in the alleys, in the attic,
in the Caves and Walrus hide.
You can wear it like the Wolf pelt or the Crane skin or your own
skin.
Best your own skin—

—it's the only thing can never be denied.

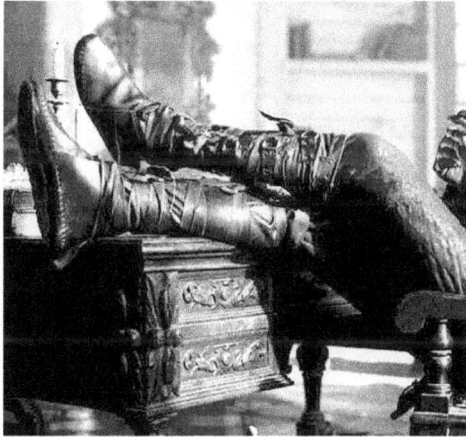

AND AIN'T THAT THE TRUTH

SCRIBBLES AND THINKING DOODLES

OR TEAR IT OUT IF YOU READ THE BACK OF A BOOK
FIRST. USE AS A PLACE-MARKER.

Abdominals – belly (dantian) muscles

Aerobic – using oxygen in a cardio-vascular workout to raise your body temperature, hence your metabolism by high-speed training; strengthens the heart, lungs, vascular system; dance, circuit, bicycling, running, boxing, martial arts, etc. are all aerobic

Alternating – one after the other

Anabolic – applies to the way in which you help your body to grow through adequate fuel and rest (it's the process whereby food is built up into protoplasm)

Anaerobic – Explains the use of oxygen in resistance training (in difference to aerobic); which is basically restrained, or forced, breathing. In other words, you don't pant when you do a lift, you force the breath out slowly on the exertion

Barbell – a long bar to which you add weight plates

B.C.A.A.'s – Branch chain amino acids

Biceps – the two muscles on the inside of the upper part of the arm

Bi's – abbr. of biceps

Buddy – another person who's also training in the same kind of routine as you and who wants to team up and work what's called set-for-set, which means that your rest between sets is equal to their set-time. Also, you can spot for each other, and encourage or correct each other. You can bounce off each other to power out the work

Burn-sets – when you want a good burn to the muscle on one of your play weeks try using a lighter weight than usual and taking the reps to the limit

Catabolize – you cannibalize, or devour, your own muscle when you over-train and under-eat

Carbohydrates – *the overall term for both simple and complex sugars/starches introduced into the body from certain foods*

Carbs – carbohydrates

Cardiovascular – the blood and heart system

Catabolic – A destructive process (opposite to anabolic) that engenders the breaking down of muscle. Happens when one over-trains (see catabolize)

Dantian – loosely translated as *elixir field*. Described as an important focal point for internal meditative techniques

Dual – both arms, or legs simultaneously

Dumbbells – hand weights

Ectomorph – (*vata* in Ayurvedic terminology) characterizes a naturally (born-that-way) lean body structure

Endomorph – (*peta* in Ayurvedic terminology) characterizes a naturally (born-that-way) medium-to-solid body structure

Endorphin – a neurologically-produced, pain-controlling, relaxant chemical; the result of the nervous system registering physical stress

Etiquette – the gyms all have an etiquette that needs to be understood, like you don't talk to someone when they're in the middle of a set; you don't go jumping onto the equipment that someone else may be using – check around first – you'll usually know because the person using that equipment will have left the plates on or some of their possessions around. You do your workout without invading the area of another person. If you need a spot you find your 'mark' (someone who knows what they're doing from your observation, or a staff member) and ask politely. If you happen to really get stuck at some point and haven't lined up a spotter it's okay to yell for help, someone always comes – same with you, if you see someone else in trouble

Extensions – from the bent position to the straight position

EZ-curl bar – a bendy bar that has weight-plates at either end, good for certain exercises

Failure – the admirable for being unable, despite extreme effort, to complete s final rep

Hydration – adequate water ingested throughout the day

Lactic acid – produced as the muscle exerts itself (that's what causes the burning sensation after an exertion). Do not have this trapped in your body. That's why you pause from 20 second to a minute between sets. Rest allows the lactic acid to settle. Anti-oxidants stabilize any potential damage from free-radicals that lactic acid is likely to generate. Lactic acid can also damage joints, so remember to rest

Mesomorph – (*kapha* in Ayurvedic terminology) a naturally (born-that-way) heavy-set body structure

Mitochondria – the 'furnace' within each cell that requires fueling from carbohydrates

Plates – the round weights that go on the ends of the bars

Preacher bench – a seat with an upper arm support in that aids you with biceps curl exercises

Program – you record the day, muscle-group, exercise, weight, number of sets, number of reps

Protein – the building blocks of the body. Without adequate protein you will not grow – it's what the body takes from certain foods specifically flesh like meat, chicken and fish

Pyramiding – is when you begin an exercise with a relatively light weight and keep adding the plates until you can only pull out 1 or 2 or 3 reps. Best done with a spotter

Spotter – someone in the gym who is willing to assist you in taking out that extra 1 or 2 reps. A good spotter is a rare and lovely being, let me tell you. They WON'T take the weight for you. They'll simply and gently assist you to get over the stuck-spot or they'll help you rack the bar when you can't, just can't get it back for yourself

Strip-sets – the opposite of pyramiding. Like burn-sets

Supplementation – the process of ingesting a manufactured relative to food when sufficient quantities of certain vitamin and minerals are missing from one's eating regime

LY DE ANGELES'S (LORE) WEBSITE
www.loredeangeles.com

RECIPE BLOG
SAVAGE
LIVING GRAIN AND SUGAR-FREE
www.almostpaleocooking.wordpress.com
For a full range of recipes and associated information

LY'S IAIDO DOJO, BYRON BAY
http://www.yaseinoshikaiaido.com.au/

YOUTUBE
https://www.youtube.com/@loredeangeles

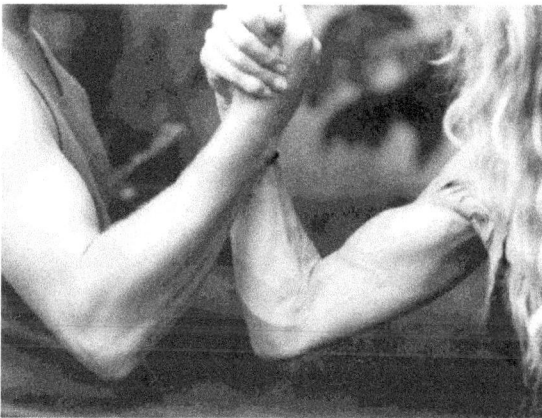

Ly and son, 1996—Image by Miriam Watson

NOTES—

remember
why you
started.

NOTES—

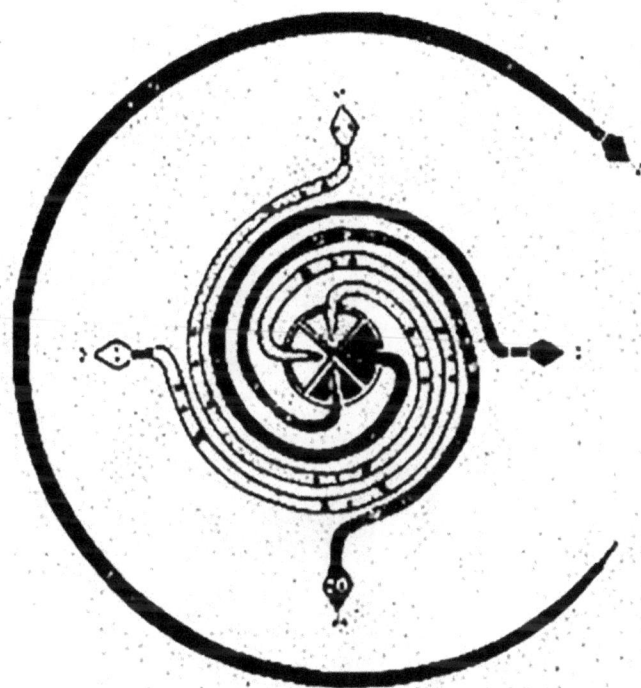

NOTES—

TEAR THIS SPARE PAGE OUT IF YOU FEEL LIKE IT—

My thanks to Melanie Spears (Brumby Books) for advice and comments on presentation of both the narrative and cover art.